The 10-Hour Coffee Diet:

Transform Your Body & Health Using 3 Weird Coffee Weight Loss Tricks!

Jennifer Jolan

and

Rich Bryda

Published by MakeRight Publishing, Inc.

ISBN: 1535274697
ISBN-13: 978-1535274692

TABLE OF CONTENTS

COPYRIGHT AND TRADEMARK NOTICES

This book is written as a source of information only. The information contained in this book should by no means be considered a substitute for the advice of a qualified medical professional, who should always be consulted before beginning any new diet, exercise, or other health program. Following the dietary instructions in this book may impact the effect of certain types of medication. Any changes in your dosage should be made only in cooperation with your prescribing physician. Before using any of the products listed in this book be sure to consult with the appropriate health professionals and check the product's label for any warnings or cautionary notes. Keep in mind that supplements are not as strictly regulated as drugs. This program is not recommended to women who are pregnant or nursing.

Products, trademarks, and trademark names are used throughout this book to describe and inform the reader about various products that are owned by third parties. No endorsement of the information contained in this book is given or implied by the owners.

All efforts have been made to ensure the accuracy of the information contained in this book as of the date published. The publisher and the authors disclaim any liability directly or indirectly from the use of the material in this book by any person.

Section 1:

The 10-Hour Coffee Diet: Transform Your Body & Health Using 3 Weird Coffee Weight Loss Tricks!

INTRODUCTION

Welcome to the 10-Hour Coffee Diet.

Over the past couple of years this diet has been tested, refined, and perfected by hundreds of different people. The diet's goal was to create a simple weight loss diet that you could do daily without it feeling like you're actually dieting. The end result grew into a diet where you lose weight effortlessly even though you're allowed to eat your favorite foods and drink plenty of coffee daily. On top of that, you won't feel miserable or hungry while on this diet. You'll actually feel awesome!

Yes, this truly is possible. Yes, you truly will get rid of belly fat.

The 10-Hour Coffee Diet is a true breakthrough in dieting. You'll simply be amazed after doing it a few times. Not only that, but you'll be able to comfortably and safely do the diet (on and off... mostly on) for the rest of your life. The best part... you get to drink lots of coffee!

This is NOT a one-size-fits-all diet. There is built-in flexibility that allows you to adjust it to your lifestyle and goals. A lot of diets require you to spend a lot of time in the kitchen making elaborate meals... not this one. A lot of diets require you to spend a lot of money... not this one.

This Diet *Is* Different

Here, you never worry about counting calories. Forget about wasting time figuring out the statistics of carbohydrates to fats to proteins and then try to fit the required amounts of all three into each day. None of that is needed for the 10-Hour Coffee Diet.

Just forget about the idea of doing a traditional diet. This isn't a traditional diet.

Follow the 10-Hour Coffee Diet for the next month (or as long as you want; there's nothing inherently unsafe about it) and you'll lose a lot of weight without much hassle. In fact, I'll bet that there's a good chance you're going to actually *enjoy following* this diet plan and continue doing it even after you lose all the weight you wanted to lose.

Most people who reach their goal weight continue doing the diet. Why? It's because they love it, it's healthy, it's simple and convenient to do, they save money, and a whole host of other reasons. You'll see what I mean after you've tried it out.

If after reading this book you don't believe the 10-Hour Coffee Diet will work for you, then all I ask is that you prove me wrong by trying it out for a week or two. Just keep an open mind and put it to a test.

I sincerely believe two weeks is enough time for you to see results that *WOW* your friends (and you) and make you a believer.

Okay, let's get you started on your weight loss journey…

1
COFFEE: THE FOUNDATION OF THE 10-HOUR COFFEE DIET

Obviously the very foundation of the 10-Hour Coffee Diet is the coffee itself.

Even if you are not now a coffee drinker, you can be successful losing weight with the 10-Hour Coffee Diet. Coffee has special properties that lend itself well to this method of fat loss. Having been around for centuries, coffee's a drink that's been consumed for so long it's a staple item of most nations. Even the tea-drinking British like a good coffee and Starbucks cafes do well in England.

Note: If you really prefer tea over coffee, you're not alone. You will see later how to adapt the 10-Hour Coffee Diet into a tea-based plan. The tea version will not be quite as effective, but in general you'll see great results.

Knowing some things about coffee, its origins, and the way people drink it will give you a good base to form the style that suits you best before you begin the 10-Hour Coffee Diet. Whether you are a coffee lover or not, you might find it interesting to learn more about the little coffee bean that makes its way from South America, Indonesia, and African nations before being ground up into your cup of water that makes the coffee you consume.

People have strong feelings about that dark caffeinated java drink called coffee. Coffee drinkers almost universally will tell you how much they love their coffee. Opinions vary on which kind of coffee is considered "best." The coffee varieties are so plentiful they can be overwhelming. Your options are almost endless.

I find that a background on how coffee went from another nation's farm to your cup may be of interest so I want to give you that background. It may encourage you to seek other options to improve upon the taste you already love.

Coffee's Evolution and Today's Ubiquitous Coffee Bars

The drink called coffee consists of water and coffee beans ground into a near-powder form. Those coffee beans grow, are harvested, dried, roasted, ground, and combined with water to form the drink. Milk, sugar, flavors, roasting methods, and brewing procedures, all go into making one coffee taste different from another.

Coffee has gone through several evolutions throughout civilization. Advances in the 1950s actually set the taste and quality of coffee back while at the same time putting it into more people's hands. Percolators were affordable by most families and pre-ground regular, and instant, and de-caffeinated coffees began lining the store shelves, not just in America, but also worldwide.

The problem with this modernized use of coffee is that coffee moved from becoming a rich, aromatic almost ritualized drink perfected by Turks, Greeks, and the Italians, to a staple item at the breakfast table. Most people considered all coffee to be the same because for most people their coffee options *were* the same.

Only recently has coffee returned to being viewed as a drink with an extra-special possibility of high quality taste. That's why so many coffee bars have sprung up around the world. Before the early 1990s, Italy was the only place where a coffee bar resided on every corner, but now most cities in America and nearly every other developed nation have them too.

> **Note:** Many of today's coffee lovers call themselves "coffee snobs" – and we're actually proud of that name!

Look just about anywhere in any town of any size in America and the chances are good you'll see a Starbucks. Sometimes, self-proclaimed coffee snobs often look upon Starbucks with disdain. They say that the Starbucks brew offers little innovation or attention to the specialized small-production variety of coffees that the world has to offer.

There is some truth to the fact that Starbucks doesn't necessarily strive to have the highest quality coffee around. But in order to have a presence in so many places around the world, Starbucks has to standardize their coffee and brew methods. This rarely pleases the self-proclaimed coffee snobs. Plus Starbucks is considered far too pricey for people who think a cup of coffee ought to cost 75-cents at the local diner.

There is a large middle ground, probably close to the majority of coffee drinkers today, who see Starbucks as sort of an oasis in life as they stop there daily to get their cups filled. In addition, the self-proclaimed coffee snobs appreciate Starbucks for opening the door for more costly, but far better quality coffees to appear. Many coffee bars today in America, for example, would have never been successful if Starbucks hadn't paved the way for premium priced, premium-flavored coffee.

> **Note:** The highest quality of coffee, no matter the form you drink it (espresso, cappuccino, latte, and so on) is universally called *specialty coffee*. Specialty coffee is served in coffee bars that take care to use only the highest quality coffee beans and brewing methods. By its very nature, a company such as Starbucks cannot offer this specifically defined "specialty coffee" because the economies of scale simply don't allow it. Plus, the highest quality of coffee comprises a small amount of coffee grown. There cannot be enough specialty coffee growers in the world to supply specialty coffee for every coffee drinker.

Is the World Crazy?

If you've been thrilled with a cheap cup of Folgers from that can sitting on your shelf for months, all this talk about coffee qualities may surprise you. You also might cringe that people expect too much from their coffee. And almost certainly you think people pay too much for "quality specialty coffee" that to you is only slightly better… maybe. But that's all good! This is why they say "variety is the spice of life." To each his, or her, own.

If you've never cared for the taste of coffee, you should consider trying it once more; not your local diner's brew though. Today's rich assortment of coffees varies vastly from your father's percolator-produced cup of coffee. And Starbucks might not be the best place to visit if you've not cared for coffee in the past due to Starbuck's fairly strong and somewhat oily flavor.

Instead you as a non-coffee drinker have many opportunities to try a rich assortment of specialty coffees, whose origins vary from all across the globe and whose method of brew can be one of ten or more methods all available at the same coffee bar. The chances that a non-coffee drinker can become a coffee lover are high today because of the quality all around us.

If you run across a coffee bar in your area that roasts its own beans, you almost certainly have found a winner! While their resulting coffee may not be your preference of taste, you can at least be assured that they strive to produce a high quality, specialty cup of coffee. These roasting coffee bars typically buy coffee beans green, freshly picked and dried, and roast coffee once or twice weekly to maintain a fresh supply. Coffee goes old quickly. Roasted coffee beans over ten days old begin to go stale. These specialty coffee bars that do their own roasting attempt to keep only the freshest beans available, both to sell in bean form for those who like specialty coffee at home and to their coffee-drinking customers who stop in for a cup.

Remember: 54% of Americans over 18 drink coffee every day[1]. 150 million people can't all be wrong! And 68% of coffee drinkers have their first cup within one hour of waking up.

Coffee Flavors High and Low

The biggest factor that goes into how a coffee in your cup tastes is the origin of the bean itself. Coffee that is grown in mountainous regions tends to have more of a fruity flavor. Coffee that is grown in lower altitudes tends to have more of a nutty flavor.

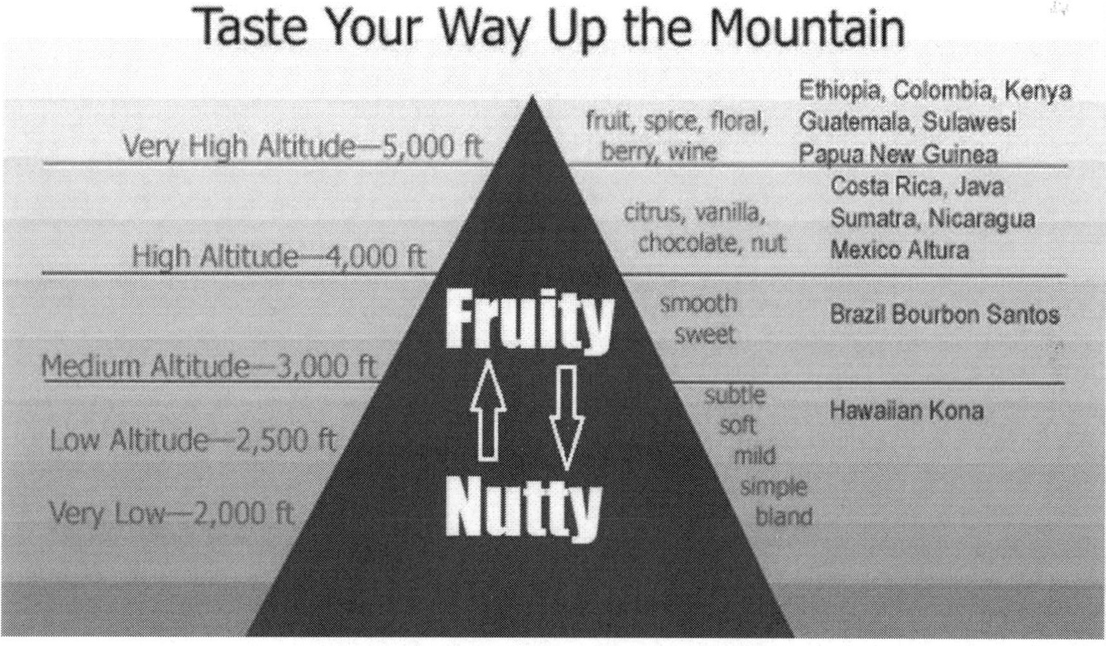

A famous but somewhat inexpensive line of coffee, Folgers, advertises itself as "Mountain Grown." This tagline implies that coffee grown at higher regions tends to be a higher quality of bean. This isn't necessarily the case for a number of reasons. High quality coffee beans can be grown at lower altitudes, producing rich nutty flavors that some people prefer over the more fruity flavors grown in higher regions.

Whether a consumer considers a specific coffee "good" is as much a matter of preference and taste as anything else. In addition, higher quality coffees tend to have more care taken during the picking, roasting, and brewing that determines whether the consumer will enjoy a cup or not. For example, if the beans are smashed and broken during their harvest, drying, or roasting, bitterness can enter the coffee flavor. The more expensive coffee beans often are more costly because of the care used in harvesting and preparing the beans.

Back to the "Mountain Grown" tagline: The altitude at which the coffee grows doesn't determine the quality in the cup. The altitude only determines a coffee bean's initial flavor.

Roasters can add flavoring during a coffee bean's roasting process. Also, *Baristas* – those who serve coffee in coffee bars – can add flavor syrups, such as hazelnut cream, to brewed coffee. You as the coffee consumer can add flavors through various syrups and creamery flavorings available. But to a coffee professional, those add-on flavors have nothing to do with a coffee bean's actual flavor. The fruity and nutty flavors determined at the coffee's original growing altitude form what is considered a coffee's true flavor and is known as the *tone* or *note* of the coffee bean in the vernacular.

So, coffee grown at higher altitudes has fruity tones and coffee grown at lower altitudes have nuttier tones.

Note: Interestingly, these are literal tones. That is, you actually can taste blueberry and other fruity flavors in high-altitude coffee. The coffee plant's roots at those high altitudes must stretch far down into the soil to get nutrients. Along the way they pick up tones of berries, even in places where those berries have never been grown! Lower altitude coffees produce a drink that you literally can taste and smell nuts, such as pecans or walnuts, as you drink your coffee.[2]

The Cloud Behind the Silver Lining: Side Effects of Caffeine

One reason non-coffee drinkers hesitate to start consuming coffee is a fear of its side effects. Coffee contains caffeine, which is a stimulant. Many coffee drinkers are truly addicted to the caffeine. Although there are far unhealthier vices, an addiction to caffeine in coffee (and tea) is real and can manifest itself both physically and psychologically.

Professor Roland Griffiths of the Johns Hopkins School of Medicine demonstrated that people who take in as little as 100 mg of caffeine daily, about the amount in a regular cup of coffee, can acquire a physical dependence that produces withdrawal symptoms which include:

- Headaches
- Muscle pain and stiffness
- Lethargy
- Nausea
- Vomiting
- Depression
- Irritability[3]

These signs can appear within 12 to 24 hours after the cessation of coffee and can last as many as nine days after withdrawing from caffeine. If you then start drinking coffee but you limit your intake, the addiction is not guaranteed to return. But if you repeat the same quantities over time, the effects will return and you can once again adopt some of the addictive traits.

Note: More than 300 mg, or three cups of coffee, over a long period of time can cause intoxicating effects that overstimulate the nervous system, flush your face, and even cause a rapid heartbeat that can result in rambling thoughts and slurred speech, not unlike intoxication through alcohol.

Certainly most people don't show signs of intoxication after three cups of coffee. But the fact that *some* do means that one should always be on the lookout for the side effects. Cut back if those side effects manifest in ways you don't want.

It's all perspective. Anything that requires your body to fight, such as caffeine-induced muscle stiffness, takes away resources from your body's full capacity performance at healthy living. Your body needs a good number of resources to fight infection, digest food properly, produce needed hormones, rid and detoxify poisons, move, sleep, talk, think, and everything else you do from day to day.

When you add an addiction into the mix you make it more difficult for your body to perform optimally. This means that too much caffeine can somewhat hinder your body's ability to lose fat and gain muscle. Then again, even a low level addiction to coffee, as many fully-functioning people have today, will not necessarily cause any adverse side effects or reduce the effectiveness of your weight loss through the 10-Hour Coffee Diet or any other diet you try.

In addition, I am somewhat biasing you early against coffee by discussing the side effects before the health benefits that coffee brings to your system. At this point if you're a coffee drinker, don't stop based on what you've read so far. And if you're not a coffee drinker, don't keep avoiding it just because of its possible side effects.

There's another side of the coin.

The Health Benefits of Coffee

As a lover of coffee, I'd never let you leave this chapter about coffee without touting its beneficial and, yes, *healthful* impact on your body. As with most things, "nothing in excess" seems to work well for coffee. You can get all of coffee's benefits without experiencing the side effects.

This means if you don't drink coffee now, you can drink it in moderation without taking on the side effects that an addiction would produce. Although coffee can be an acquired taste, people who doubt they will like the flavor often quickly learn that coffee can be one of the most enjoyable drinks available. As mentioned earlier, if you've tried coffee in the past and didn't care for it, you should consider trying coffee once more... the 10-Hour Coffee Diet way.

Massive Antioxidants in Every Cup

Antioxidants are enemies of free radicals in your body. Free radicals are thieves. They steal stable molecules' electrons from your body. This is a normal process of living and aging. Still, free radicals cause damage to cells over time in numbers that can cause problems in your body. While there is no way to eliminate this, antioxidants fight the effects of cell damage done by free radicals.

According to one study in 2005, there is "nothing close" to coffee that provides as many antioxidants for your body's well-being[4]. In addition to having loads of these cancer-resistant and age-prolonging antioxidants, the antioxidants in fruits and vegetables don't seem to be absorbed by our bodies as well as the antioxidants in coffee. Perhaps that's due to coffee providing them in a liquid form and getting those needed nutrients to our cells more quickly. In doing this, your healthy cells stay healthy longer and are damaged less. Toxins have more difficulty remaining in your system because your waste disposal mechanisms work best with reduced free radicals that drain your body's resources.

Stress Less by Smelling More

Can't sleep? Coffee certainly won't help on that front, but if you are tired from too-little sleep, researchers at the Seoul National University[5] actually discovered that sleep-deprived rats *only had to smell coffee* and they'd begin producing brain proteins that deal well with sleep-deprived stress.

The morning smell of coffee brewing truly does give you a morning pick-me-up by stimulating some good proteins to help you through the morning.

Coffee Can Help with the Effects of Alcohol

Liver failure is a common side effect of drinking too much alcohol over a long period of time. *Liver cirrhosis* develops in people who drink too much alcohol. Liver cirrhosis is an autoimmune disease that can result in both cancer and liver failure.

A single daily cup of coffee, however, can shield many against liver cirrhosis.[6] Obviously you don't want to use coffee as a crutch to go wild on alcohol, but even non-alcoholics may find a healthier liver as they age if they drink coffee. The association between coffee and a healthier liver cannot be ignored. Especially when the Duke-NUS Graduate Medical School found that drinking four or more cups of coffee daily could help prevent non-alcoholic fatty liver disease (NAFLD).[7]

Happiness is a Warm Cup

Although an addiction can occur with only a few cups, four or more cups daily provide benefits to your well-being. (Life's full of trade-offs, especially with coffee!)

The National Institute of Health determined that people who drank at least four cups of coffee daily had lower rates of depression than people who don't drink coffee.[8] This depression wasn't connected to the caffeine either. The lower depression numbers didn't correlate with Coke, which also has caffeine. Coke, they stated, as opposed to coffee, actually increased depression factors in its drinkers.

The NIH's specific conclusion was this:

> *This large prospective study suggests that frequent consumption of diet-sweetened beverages may increase depression risk among older adults, whereas coffee consumption may lower the risk.*

Related to these findings, the Harvard School of Public Health found that coffee drinkers – all other factors being equal – had a lower rate of suicide than those who drink fewer than two cups daily. The mild antidepressant in coffee stimulates your body's own "happy" neurotransmitters such as serotonin, dopamine, and noradrenaline.[9] These findings were quite astonishing when one learns that the Harvard School of Public Health determined that two or more cups daily can decrease the suicide risk by *as much as 50 percent.*

> **Note:** You'll learn all about these brain neurotransmitters and how to maximize them in the second section of this book.

Parkinson's Patients Find Relief in Java

Victims of Parkinson's disease find that their symptoms are lessened when they drink coffee. Ronald Postuma, M.D., of Science Daily, recently reported that not only are people who drink coffee less likely to develop Parkinson's disease, but that the caffeine in coffee helps with the movement problems that Parkinson's patients often experience.[10]

Help for Type 2 Diabetes Risk

The American Chemical Society's researchers found that those who drink four or more cups of coffee daily reduce their Type 2 diabetes risk by as much as 50 percent.[11] For those of us who really love the stuff, there's even better news that came out of that study: for each *additional* daily cup, your chance of developing Type 2 diabetes lowers another 7 percent!

Female Skin Cancer Countered

Skin cancer has been a growing problem for the past 40 years or so, especially due to the now-determined bad advice to avoid the sun and its vitamin D3. There are discussions underway to put labels on sunscreen, warning against their overuse after decades of saying the opposite. It turns out that people today get far too little vitamin D3, a vitamin that used to be in ample supply for most of us who got regular sun exposure.

Not only does adequate exposure to the sun actually appear to *reduce* skin cancer, as you probably guessed by now, so does coffee. At least coffee apparently reduces skin cancer in females who drink three or more cups daily. Harvard Medical School conducted an 112,897-person study along with the Brigham and Women's Hospital over 20 years and their findings are welcome results for female coffee drinkers.[12]

For Brain *and* Brawn

Coffee keeps your brain healthier *and* makes you a better athlete!

Alzheimer's disease is a growing problem, but it grows more slowly in coffee drinkers according to a combined study lead by the University of South Florida and the University of Miami.[13] They found that regular coffee consumption helped reduce the chance of Alzheimer's and kept the brains healthier. Those who did develop Alzheimer's did so later than the non-coffee drinkers, as many as four years later.

In addition, coffee makes you smarter!

CNN's health website explained how coffee makes you much sharper if you're sleep-deprived.[14] We all should get plenty of sleep, but at times life doesn't allow us to get a lot of sleep due to a deadline or other activities. Time Reporter Michael Lemonick explained that sleep deprived coffee drinkers experience a surge of several mental activities including:

- Speed of reaction
- Attention span
- Logic and reasoning
- Reaction time

Coffee improves not only the brain's performance, but also your body's overall performance. The New York Times recently reported that a pre-workout or pre-event cup of coffee enhances an athlete's performance. This is due to the increased number of fatty acids that enter the bloodstream from coffee drinking. Those fatty acids enable muscles to absorb and burn those fats for fuel more readily than they could otherwise do.[15]

Your Remedy: Drink Coffee

And remember, not only does coffee help with the health effects above, you're about to experience one of the most unusual and most effective fat-loss diets you've ever seen... and its centerpiece is going to be a good ol' cup of coffee.

So, the next time someone reminds you of the side effects to caffeine, you remind *them* that good coffee, made right and in moderation, can be just what the doctor ordered!

Coffee Making Methods

Many of us enjoy coffee, and sometimes tea, and one of the reasons those appeal to us, other than their health benefits, is the number of ways we can drink them.

Here's just a short list, far from complete, of the more common ways used to prepare coffee and tea:

- Iced tea
- Hot tea
- Sun tea
- Coffee (hot, made from a drip process or percolator, the most common and generic form of coffee served in America)
- Iced coffee
- Espresso (typically served in a small 1- or 2-ounce demitasse cups made from strongly-flavored, dark-roasted coffee beans)
- Cappuccino (one part espresso, one part hot milk, and one part steamed milk called the "froth")
- Pour over (found in many of the more advanced coffee bars today where water for coffee is poured over a thin filter directly into the cup for immediate drinking)
- French press (hot water manually pushed tightly through a filtering glass tube)

That list doesn't include the myriad of flavorings and milks and creams we can add to produce an array of flavor combinations we will never grow tired of. Not only do we have an extremely wide assortment of methods to make coffee, there is an even wider assortment of coffees to choose from.

Note: If you're an espresso drinker, you can make the 10-Hour Coffee Diet's coffee using espresso! You must turn it into an *Americano*, which is simple to do. You'll see how to make the coffee using espresso when we get to that chapter.

Surprisingly, the coffees that people assume have higher levels of caffeine, don't. Dark roasts and espresso coffees actually are some of the weakest when it comes to caffeine levels. In general, the darker and stronger the roast or brewing method, the *less* caffeine it will have. This isn't always true because coffee made at Starbucks is fairly dark and strong and it has some of the highest caffeine levels you can consume.

But in general, don't be afraid of trying the darker roasts and methods such as espresso if you previously thought they'd have more caffeine. Sourcing your own coffee and making it at home not only saves you money, but you will almost always be able to make a better tasting coffee than just about any place else – with the possible exception of local specialty coffee bars with the highest of standards and trained Baristas.

In 2010, the *Journal of Food Science* published this list of types of coffee and the caffeine levels each has and the results might surprise you:[16]

Type of coffee	Size	Caffeine
Espresso, coffee-bar style	1 oz. (30 mL)	40-75 mg
Generic brewed	8 oz. (240 mL)	95-200 mg
Generic instant	8 oz. (240 mL)	27-173 mg
McDonald's brewed	16 oz. (480 mL)	100 mg
McDonald's Mocha Frappe	16 oz. (480 mL)	125 mg
Starbucks Latte	16 oz. (480 mL)	150 mg
Starbucks Pike Place brewed	16 oz. (480 mL)	330 mg

Note: Some larger "dessert coffee drinks" such as Frappes contain more calories than a fully loaded cheeseburger and fries. Be careful that you limit these drinks to extremely rare occasions. They can too easily skyrocket your blood sugar and greatly speed fat gain.

The coffee ritual is just as important as the taste for some of us more hardcore java drinkers. The ritual of making it, using some of the more creative ways, is half the fun... and the other half is seeking ways to perfect your next cup so it's just a little richer, better tones, and a higher quality texture than the last one.

What Kind of Coffee to Try?

It's impossible to tell you the kind of coffee you'll like. As with ice cream, "to each his (or her) own."

A few factors go into finding one you like however. If you're a coffee snob already, there's little I can tell you that you don't already do to excess – as do I.

Before I take a quick tour of how to improve the taste and quality of the coffee you drink, let me state: Coffee is grown using an extremely high amount of pesticides. Consider drinking organic coffee that doesn't have this problem. I discuss this in more depth later.

If you are a coffee drinker but would like to improve upon the taste and experience some of the better specialty coffees out there, you're in for an endless journey finding just the right taste for you. It's a fun trip. One of the ways you will immediately begin improving your coffee is to follow some of the guidelines I point out below.

If you've never liked coffee, or simply never gotten accustomed to it, following these simple guidelines will help steer you in a direction where you can find the perfect brew for you.

- Consider avoiding pre-ground coffee. Oxygen begins to oxidize (destroy) coffee the moment roasted beans are exposed to the air. This means starting from the moment they are picked from the coffee plant overseas they begin to deteriorate, but the deterioration process speeds up considerably once beans exit the roaster. The oldest coffee you can buy is pre-ground because it *is* turning rancid before it hits your cup. This leads right into the next tip. Rancid doesn't mean dangerous, but you won't get as rich of taste if you buy pre-ground. Again, you decide what is best for *you,* but consider trying an option other than pre-ground to see how you like it. To some, the cost and effort isn't worth it... and that's fine.

- Instead of pre-ground, you can buy whole coffee beans. Oxygen destroys coffee even in its bean form. But in its original bean form the interior of the bean takes longer to break down and longer to begin getting rancid due to oxygen exposure.
- When possible and if you don't mind spending more, buy only local, fresh whole coffee beans. Keep the coffee in its bean form until you're ready for a cup. This means that you want to grind your coffee beans right before you make coffee. This means those beans are bought as soon as possible after the beans were roasted. If a local coffee bar roasts its own beans, you have the *best* chance of getting fresh, non-rancid coffee beans. Coffee in bags on grocery store shelves generally have sat too long, even in an well-sealed package, to be considered good enough to drink according to most coffee professionals. But again, you are the master of your coffee destiny, so it's all up to you on what you decide.

Note: Large coffee companies add flavoring and preservatives during the roasting process so they can sell vast amounts of coffee, even in bean form, without the rancid taste coming through to the cup. This is why pre-ground coffee used by your mother for her percolator never *tasted* rancid.

- Fresh can be too fresh! If a local coffee shop roasts its own beans, you're on your way to a great cup of coffee. Still, the freshly roasted coffee beans should have a couple of days after roasting to settle. This enables the roasting flavors to combine and gives the roasted beans time to prepare for grinding. So find out what day your coffee bar roasts its beans, and pick up a bag a couple of days later. If you happen to pick it up on roasting day or the next day, just keep it sealed in the bag for a couple of days after that before you use the beans for coffee.
- Keep all unused coffee, pre-ground or beans, in an airtight container. Used to be we were told to keep coffee in the refrigerator or freezer to maintain freshness, but we know now this does the opposite. When the beans come out of cold storage, they condensate and the moisture *speeds* up their decaying process. Just get a sealable glass jar to store the beans, such as the Bormioli here: amazon.com/Bormioli-Rocco-Round-Clear-4-Ounce/dp/B0001BMYGQ
- Never store coffee beans in plastic containers.
- Coffee beans that look oily are not fresh. When a bean begins to age and go rancid, the oils are pushed out of the interior of the bean and the outside surface looks oily. It's counter-intuitive, but oily beans actually look very good because the oil literally "oils them up" and makes them shine and look fresh. The big companies know this and certainly don't mind that the old coffee beans you get at the grocery store look fresh even when the opposite is true. If you buy fresh beans and begin to see oily residue on the outside of the beans, they are turning and it's time to get a fresh supply. If you decide to keep using those oily beans, you won't notice a tremendously different flavor. Again, you make the final call.
- Well-sealed, coffee bean freshness only lasts about ten days to two weeks. If you don't make enough coffee to use up your beans in a couple of weeks, consider buying fewer beans to stay on the freshness curve.
- Try both nutty and fruity toned coffee. Your coffee bar's Barista should be able to tell you which of the shop's beans are fruity (grown at high altitudes) and which are nutty (grown at lower altitudes). Try them both. Better, over time try *all* the different roasts that your local shop provides. Some that might not have a good-sounding name may taste very good to you, so try them all before settling in on one or two favorites.

- If you decide to buy whole beans instead of pre-ground, you also must get a grinder. With it you will grind just enough beans for your next cup of coffee. If you're going to make a cup of coffee, or a pot, *that* is when you grind just enough beans for the cup or pot. This implies you need a coffee bean grinder. You can get cheap blade grinders, but coffee snobs certainly don't like the consistency of blade grinders. If you're starting out, or just experimenting to try new tastes, you don't want to spend $300 and up for a "quality" burr grinder. Feel free to get a blade grinder such as the Hamilton-Beach for under $20. You'll save money that you can use to try new roasts of coffees. (Available on Amazon at: amazon.com/Hamilton-Beach-80365-Hands-Free-Platinum/dp/B000FBYRMQ).
- Feel like experimenting? One of the most marvelous coffee inventions to come around in a long time is the cheap little *Aerobie*, also called the *AeroPress Coffee and Espresso Maker*. This is a hard plastic tube with a plunger and small filters. No electricity is needed and it's so portable, coffee snobs such as Tim Ferriss, the writer, takes one onto an airplane and makes his needed coffee sitting in his seat. There is no electricity needed and you can use pre-ground coffee or grind your beans right before you make it. Oh, and you need a hot water source. The Aerobie is also available on Amazon (at amazon.com/Aerobie-AeroPress-Coffee-Espresso-Maker/dp/B0047BIWSK). Here is what the Aerobie looks like:

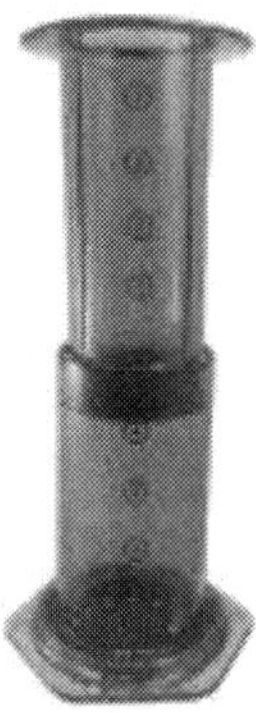

Doesn't look like much of a coffee maker, does it? The worst kept secret in the coffee industry is that Baristas at most major coffee bars, when pressured, admit they make the best coffee at home with their Aerobie and not with the $15,000 equipment in the coffee bar. Purists are beginning to admit that there is not a better method out there, or at least certainly not a method available to the common household, that makes a more perfect cup than an Aerobie. And the Aerobie comes with a bonus: complete clean up takes about 6 seconds; just try cleaning any other coffee-making equipment completely in 6 seconds!

The 10-Hour Coffee Diet (hang in there, we're getting to it) uses coffee that the Aerobie is a perfect vehicle for making. Although you have a few ways to make your 10-Hour Coffee Diet's coffee, by using an Aerobie you are most likely to get the most flavor from the fresh beans you grind over any other method.

The Aerobie isn't necessarily the best way to make a lot of coffee, such as your next three days' worth, if your job or lifestyle requires that you make several cups of coffee at once. Use a traditional Mr. Coffee-like drip coffee maker if you want to make a lot at once. Although such a device makes us coffee snobs cringe, the biggest secret to good coffee is the coffee itself, so go with a high quality coffee and grind the beans right before you brew a cup. Even the least expensive coffee makers will produce a wonderful cup as long as you use a quality roast and freshly-ground beans.

What About Decaf?

Decaffeinated coffee is not pure coffee. Coffee is only coffee when it is made from a coffee bean. Coffee beans have caffeine. The removal of the caffeine can do nothing positive for the taste or freshness of coffee.

Although, if you make decaf, you will not usually experience the addiction problems associated with too much prolonged coffee drinking. You also will lose out on some of the health benefits that the unadulterated coffee with its natural caffeine content provides. Still, there are people whose doctors have warned them off caffeine for various health reasons. Obviously you should listen to your doctor, especially if you know of a specific health condition that is adversely affected when you ingest caffeine.

If you must drink decaffeinated coffee, the 10-Hour Coffee Diet will still work almost to full capacity. You will lose some of the metabolic benefits of regular coffee, but it won't affect the diet in any extreme way. You almost certainly will find it to be one of the fastest ways to shred fat you've ever known in spite of the lack of caffeine in your coffee.

If you do want to seek out the best-tasting decaf, certainly follow all of the general quality coffee guidelines, such as buying only fresh decaffeinated beans, grinding them right before you make coffee, and so on. Just because you're not drinking the caffeine doesn't mean you should shortchange freshness and taste. But still, an inexpensive pre-ground bag of organic decaf coffee will be fine for the 10-Hour Coffee Diet if your bank account and personal preferences prefer it.

Note: If you like milk-based coffee drinks, such as cappuccino and latte, you can have all of them with decaf. The fresher and the higher quality of decaf bean you buy, the less difference you will taste between it and the caffeinated version of the same roast.

How Important is Organic?

Coffee is a product with some of the highest concentrations of pesticides. Even if you don't eat a fully organic diet, coffee is often the one time you should consider organic. Keep in mind that many of the specialty coffees that are considered the highest quality are not all organic. Still, their more manual processing and care generally means that pesticides required for their growth are far less than conventional non-organic coffees.

If you buy beans online or from a grocery store, instead of from a specialty coffee bar, you actually might find organic coffee that is a higher quality coffee than the standard grocery fare, but is less costly than the specialty coffees. Certainly that is fine, especially if finances dictate that you don't spend money on a specialty coffee at a local coffee bar. But if you do buy in a grocery store and don't mind spending a little more, try to stick to the higher quality stores such as Whole Foods. And look for organic coffee roasts above everything else when you do.

Online at Amazon, consider using Cameron's coffee brand here: amazon.com/Camerons-Organic-French-Coffee-32-Ounce/dp/B002ESSASK

Cameron's also makes a pre-ground organic coffee. You'll find all their varieties on Amazon.

Note: If you're in the UK you can probably find most or all of these products listed on the Amazon.co.uk website. If you're not in the USA or UK, check your national Amazon website (if you have one) or you can search online or go to a local health food store. Unfortunately, prices vary around the world on products from country to country, even after taking exchange rates into consideration. So you'll have to adjust my price calculations as needed.

Since coffee is the cornerstone for this book, I'd like to offer one additional option other than Cameron's because this one offers a very different, more fruity tone and you may prefer it over the Cameron's one. Seattle's Best makes high quality roasted coffee, one of the best blends we've tried for the price, and you can be assured it's as fresh as possible. Even their pre-ground is packed quickly after roasting and is about as fresh as pre-ground can be. Plus, you get the convenience of not having to grind your beans while still getting an organic coffee.

Seattle's Best organic pre-ground coffee is available on Amazon here: amazon.com/Seattles-Best-Coffee-Organic-Ground/dp/B002HQBWLQ/

Although some specialty coffees are certainly overpriced, in *general* the more you pay, the higher the quality.

Your local coffee bar, if a specialty coffee shop, may roast its own beans and source from a single coffee plantation that the owner controls. This is fairly common these days in larger cities. Even in many medium-sized cities you can find coffee bars that follow the coveted *Seed to Cup* method of controlling the entire coffee-growing process. With Seed to Cup, the owners of your coffee bar actually owns a portion of the coffee plantation and is able to control the quality of the production of the beans. In your town or as you travel, ask if the coffee bar utilizes the Seed to Cup. If it does, you are in for one of the most amazing coffees you've ever imagined.

2
"HOW FAST?"

The 10-Hour Coffee Diet contains an important element that amplifies its ability to shred the fat from your thighs, hips, and belly. That vital element is *intermittent fasting.*

Fasting is a time period in which you do not eat any food. Various forms of fasting exist, some allow for juice such as lemon juice only. Water is almost always allowed and there's no way you should consider a fast that includes no water without your doctor's order.

Intermittent fasting is a type of fast where you don't go entire 24-hour time periods without food. In other words, every 24 hours you eat something. You just don't eat your usual 3 or 4 meals a day with snacks in-between.

Intermittent fasting is what we'll concern ourselves with here, not traditional fasting for long periods of time. While some people may fast for multiple 24-hour time periods for spiritual or health reasons, that isn't anything close to what you'll do on the 10-Hour Coffee Diet. The intermittent fast you perform on the 10-Hour Coffee Diet is simple and almost everybody finds it easy to maintain. Hunger won't even be an issue.

The premise of this diet is to do a mini, modified fast. This will be the intermittent fasting that you will do. Again, *you should find it to be simple.* You will not have to be on an intermittent fast every day of the week, although many of us find that it becomes routine and our bodies respond better when we stay on some form of an intermittent fast every day.

Fear Not the Fast

Don't let the term *fast* frighten you away from the 10-Hour Coffee Diet. It can't be repeated enough, the kind of fast you undergo on the 10-Hour Coffee Diet is a simple one. Many people find that they adapt to it within two to four days and some immediately take to it the first day and never look back. It's most interesting to find that those who begin intermittent fasting, again fasting that lasts less than 24 hours, often have absolutely *no* trouble with hunger during the fasting hours.

Your results should not be much different from most other people.

An intermittent fast usually begins from before you go to bed at night and ends the next day sometime. The hours after your last meal before bedtime combined with the eight or so hours you sleep comprise the bulk of your fast. This is why most people feel no loss when they begin an intermittent fasting program. The end of your intermittent fast will be sometime *after* the traditional early breakfast ("break fast") time.

The intermittent fasting benefits of the 10-Hour Coffee Diet produces one of the most effective fat-loss programs available.

> **Note:** If the very thought of fasting causes your stomach to rumble and you start to feel the "fight or flight" response to this entire book, you're in good company! Most of us are hesitant the first time any fasting option is presented. But keep reading to see how easy this whole thing is. *So* easy, in fact, it's shocking that this amazing fat-loss plan wasn't discovered long ago. Intermittent fasting almost never causes people to dream of massive holiday turkey dinners or experience nightmares of an endless line of empty plates.

Why Avoid Full Fasting

Traditional fasting that lasts for one or more 24-hour periods does provide health benefits that include advanced detoxification. Certainly weight loss occurs during full fasts, although much of that weight loss is muscle and water weight, not fat loss. Some find that they experience even a spiritual detox when they fast.

As mentioned above, fasts are well known for their ability to trigger weight loss. This weight loss can be dramatic. But if weight loss is your sole reason for going on a traditional fast, that is far from ideal. You will lose a lot of muscle, which forces your metabolism to slow down. This causes you to rebound and regain weight quickly once you begin eating again. Unfortunately, it's fat that you regain, not the muscle you lost. Often you'll regain *more* weight after a full fasting-related diet.

The Details of Full Fasting Problems

It's worth revisiting the concept of a full fast before we get more into an intermittent fast because people sometimes overdo a diet when they have reached their wit's end with fat loss. If you're like virtually everybody else, we all from time to time get desperate and go overboard in an effort to lose weight as fast as possible. You *may* be tempted to perform full fasts once you see how easy an intermittent fast can be.

Don't.

On a traditional fast where you don't eat or drink any calories, your body literally starts to cannibalize its own muscle tissues as a source of fuel. This enables you to function and survive. Your body does this because it assumes you're in a starvation mode. To survive starvation your body automatically begins to utilize muscle for fuel because you don't *have* to retain all your muscle to stay alive.

This cannibalization of your muscles, done to your body by your body, is life-extending if you're ever lost in the middle of the ocean or desert for days on end. But in normal, everyday life, it's bad. More accurately, full fasting for the sole reason of weight loss is *extremely* bad.

The reason why such a calorie-restrictive fast is bad is because muscle is more metabolically active than fat. In simple terms this means that you burn more calories to maintain a pound of muscle as compared to a pound of fat. So, during a typical fast where you don't eat or drink any calories and your body attacks muscle tissues in order for you to survive, the body essentially is down-regulating your metabolism.

Not only is muscle far superior when it comes to burning calories, muscles take up far less space in your body than fat does. A pound of fat consumes much more space in your body than does a pound of muscle... thus making you look leaner. Quality weight loss programs, such as the 10-Hour Coffee Diet, focus on *fat* loss and not *weight* loss.

When you lose muscle, your metabolism automatically slows down because you're losing metabolically active muscle tissues that burn off a lot of calories. If you lose those muscle tissues, you lose the ability to burn off more calories while at rest. Over the course of a day you burn far more calories during your at-rest periods than you do during your combined exercise and movement periods, except in extremely active cases. If you lose muscle, you lose the ability to lose fat weight and keep it off.

The Solution to Muscle Loss

Simply put, you will not have a problem with muscle loss if you follow the 10-Hour Coffee Diet. First, you will never refrain from eating as you do in full fasts. Plus, one of the primary advantages of intermittent fasting is the lack of muscle loss while promoting fat loss.

What you essentially will do is primarily feed your muscles a good fat and protein every few hours to maintain those muscles. Muscle tissue is made up of proteins. By modifying the traditional fast in this way, you spare your muscles and your body will instead burn off your body fat. Therefore, there exists absolutely no reason to burn muscle and your body is smart enough to know that.

> **Note:** Consuming fat does not make you fat. Not all fats are equal. Many fats, such as polyunsaturated fats in most fast food, are unhealthy for your body. The fats you consume on the 10-Hour Coffee Diet program will be the highest quality fats, also known as "good fats."

The Health Benefits of Intermittent Fasting

Studies abound on health benefits when we adopt an intermittent fasting lifestyle. Intermittent fasting often ends up being a lifestyle for most of those who begin such a fasting regimen. They decide that intermittent fasting isn't a temporary thing. The health benefits of intermittent fasting fully support a lifelong intermittent fasting regimen. So even if you stop following the 10-Hour Coffee Diet after you get the body you want, you may still want to maintain an intermittent fasting eating routine.

Fat loss isn't the only advantage to intermittent fasting. Intermittent fasting also improves blood lipid profiles, improves insulin sensitivity, enhances cognitive function, and a whole host of other great things. As a matter of fact, the very nature of intermittent fasting fights any muscle loss that a longer-term fast would produce because the intermittent fast increases your body's natural production of growth hormones.[17]

Heart Health

Fasting is certainly heart healthy. In 2011, the Intermountain Medical Center Heart Institute reported that fasting reduced all of these health risk factors[18]:

- Cardiac risk
- Triglycerides
- Blood sugar levels that helped regular insulin and avoid diabetes

As a bonus, the British Journal of Diabetes and Vascular Disease state the following:

> Fasting also appears to aid those with ischemic heart disease. Fasting may even protect the heart by raising levels of adiponectin, a protein that has several important roles in carbohydrate and lipid metabolism and vascular biology.[19]

Diabetes Risks Reduced

Insulin sensitivity is a major problem today. Obesity is a problem that exasperates the problem dramatically. In addition to helping you lose the fat, though, The British Journal of Diabetes and Vascular Disease study mentioned above addressed diabetes risks, especially Type 2 diabetes.

Its study concluded:

> *Scientists have known since the 1940s that intermittent fasting helps us lose weight, and can cut the incidence of diabetes in lab animals. Recent studies have also confirmed that restricting calorie intake could possibly reverse Type 2 diabetes in some people. Researchers measured improved pancreatic function and fewer of the fatty deposits associated with insulin resistance were present in fasting subjects.*

Our Meal Frequency

Three meals a day, whether we want or need them, doesn't seem to be the way our bodies were designed to get fuel. The benefits of fasting seem to imply that our bodies desire a reduced number of meals each day.

Several diet plans, some of which are successful, promote eating five or more mini-meals daily to normalize insulin and digestion and to help promote weight loss. It is beginning to be thought that such eating plans are not the reason for the weight loss. It is thought now that the *kind* of food promoted in those plans is the reason for the weight loss, not the meal frequency.

Consider what happens when you eat a big lunch and then go to a meeting at 1:00 pm. Are you alert and an active participant? Most likely the opposite is true. You are sluggish and your attention begins to drift off. Heck, you may actually fall asleep in the meeting. There is a physiological reason this occurs.

Digestion is one of the most strenuous internal activities your body performs. To digest food your body must borrow a lot of resources otherwise used for thinking, breathing, walking, talking, and so on. One of the ways your body can do this best is to slow you down. Optimally, a nap after a big meal allows your body to utilize resources most effectively and fully. While you may have been told that a long nap after a big meal increases your fat gain, there is little evidence that is true. The *type* of food you eat and when you eat it has a much greater impact on your fat levels than sleeping after a meal.

They all seem to say, "Breakfast is the most important meal of the day!"

Why?

Where are the studies? It turns out that you need your body's resources to start your day without slowing it down through digestion. During your night's sleep your body goes through all sorts of housekeeping. Not only does it digest any remaining food, but it also detoxifies itself and works on fighting excess body fat. Dr. Joel Robbins[20] states that once you awaken, your body hasn't stopped the process fully and that you need the first few hours of the day to allow it to continue. This seems to be consistent with the benefits of intermittent fasting, both as a fat-reduction process as well as a healthier way of eating.

The Department of Human Biology at the University of Limburg in The Netherlands performed a detailed study of subjects called "nibblers" who ate six small meals a day compared to those "gorgers" who ate the same food in only two meals a day. They found that the ultimate metabolic rates were identical as was their rate of *carbohydrate oxidation* (the burn rate of extra carbs).[21]

While some might see this as reason not to bother with intermittent fasting, that study differed in a major way from the way you will perform your daily intermittent fast. Both groups in that study were given the same amount and type of food in every 24-hour time period. You, however, will *not* eat the same amount of food during your non-fasting period. *More important, you will not want that much food.* You naturally want less food during your eating hours, as you will see almost immediately. Although the 10-Hour Coffee Diet's fat loss does not primarily come from the slightly less caloric intake you'll naturally get, the fewer calories help and may be one of the reasons for the improved health factors mentioned earlier.

It's been said that energy is boosted when one eats several smaller meals daily instead of two or three larger meals. This, too, seems to be nothing more than a myth that is perpetuated from dieter to dieter without any basis in fact. The Department of Nutrition and Dietetics at King's College in London studied this very thing. Did the people who ate several small meals have more energy than those who ate two or three larger meals? Is breakfast *really* the "most important meal of the day" or is the opposite actually true?

It turns out that short-term energy attributed to multi-meal eaters is the same level as that from those who fast from breakfast in the mornings and is the same level as those who eat fewer meals that are somewhat larger.[22] That study focused on extremely obese patients and a chamber calorimeter, which measures actual energy expended. They used the meter to determine their energy levels throughout each day of the study.

Note: If you are pregnant, it's suggested that you do not go on an intermittent fast until you've weaned your baby. The reasons are not yet conclusive as to how important this is because some early studies have shown mixed results. To be safe, you and your baby come first, so avoid intermittent fasting until the weaning.

Note: If you are currently hypoglycemic or a diabetic, you almost surely should work to regulate your system before beginning any intermittent fast program. This is true in spite of the fact that intermittent fasting helps your body regulate blood sugar as mentioned before. For now, depending on the severity of your situation, your insulin levels are far too precarious to mess with on your own. Consider a low-carb, high-fat (good fats such as organic cold pressed olive oil, organic virgin coconut oil, and nuts and seeds) and moderately high protein diet where you get most of your carbs from non-starchy vegetables and a small bit of berries. This diet does wonders for many people to help them begin to naturally regulate insulin problems. Your doctor, especially if you have one who is open to alternative healing options, in addition to traditional medicines, should be able to tell you when you can safely begin your intermittent fast and begin the full 10-Hour Coffee Diet.[23]

The Research Seems to Support an Easy Intermittent Fasting Experience

All of these studies support the anecdotal evidence of tens of thousands of people who routinely follow an intermittent fasting lifestyle. Your health should improve (all things being equal), your fat levels will go down, you will maintain your muscles (and metabolism), and you'll either maintain or increase your energy levels.

Note: Many see an *increase* in energy throughout the day in spite of the fact they eat less food and fast several hours more a day than they used to by sleeping through the night. It's likely that our bodies simply function better when we don't keep our digestive system working hard more hours than it was designed to work.

Keep all this in mind as you read through the rest of this book and as you learn more about the 10-Hour Coffee Diet. Eating your largest meal at night does not contribute to fat gain or energy loss, as we used to be told.

Drinks While Fasting

Non-caloric drinks are allowed during you fasting and non-fasting hours, although you'll probably want to save the coffee for its very specific and timed use in the 10-Hour Coffee Diet. Colas are almost universally frowned upon these days by health professionals, even the diet ones which are chemical factories putting nothing good into your system.

You'll drink all the water you want during fasting times. Of course the cleaner the water the better... so municipal tap water is a last choice if you have the option of using mineral water or water you run through a filter that removes chlorine and other chemicals. I'll mention a great low-cost Brita filter a little later when we discuss the water used in the 10-Hour Coffee Diet. You can spend more and get a counter filter such as the Berkey, which is one of our favorite countertop filters. You can get whole-house filters that do all sorts of powerful filtering using "reverse osmosis" but the cost escalates drastically for something like those.

Tea is an option that you can drink between 10-Hour Coffee Diet coffees and with your meals. All I ask is that if you drink tea, drink a lot of purified water to keep your system flushed and to reduce the effects of the caffeine you're getting.

Some people want to follow the 10-Hour Coffee Diet and use tea instead of coffee. This is fine! If tea is your preference, you absolutely can drink tea. You'll see how to integrate tea into the 10-Hour Coffee Diet a little later.

Your Fat Metabolizing Rate

Dr. Joseph Mercola, M.D., is a huge proponent of intermittent fasting. His conclusion about such an eating lifestyle is a good conclusion to this chapter to leave you with:

It takes about six to eight hours for your body to metabolize your glycogen stores and after that you start to shift to burning fat. However, if you are replenishing your glycogen by eating every eight hours (or sooner), you make it far more difficult for your body to use your fat stores as fuel.

It's long been known that restricting calories in certain animals can increase their lifespan by as much as 50 percent, but more recent research suggests that sudden and intermittent calorie restriction appears to provide the same health benefits as constant calorie restriction, which may be helpful for those who cannot successfully reduce their everyday calorie intake (or aren't willing to).

Unfortunately, hunger is a basic human drive that can't be easily suppressed, so anyone attempting to implement serious calorie restriction is virtually guaranteed to fail. Fortunately you don't have to deprive yourself as virtually all of the benefits from calorie restriction can be achieved through properly applied intermittent fasting.

3
THE 10-HOUR COFFEE DIET'S 3 WEIRD TRICKS

This book introduces you to individual concepts before giving you the whole, big picture. Generally, a subject is best mastered when you can see the overall nature of the topic you're studying first. Then you can dig into the nitty-gritty details.

The 10-Hour Coffee Diet is the opposite. If you got the overview first, it would raise far more questions than it answers. For example, now that you understand intermittent fasting and now that you realize the health benefits, as well as how simple it is to stay on, that aspect of the 10-Hour Coffee Diet will not be a stumbling block to you as it would have been if this book simply began with a required intermittent fast. You're far more open and even curious as to how an intermittent fast will affect you now that you understand the background.

The first chapter of this book, all about coffee, was useful to begin with for two reasons:

1. People who already love coffee never tire of learning more about their beloved beverage.
2. People who never liked the taste of coffee got an understanding of why the coffee they may have tried previously was the problem, not coffee itself. They now have several avenues to taste truly quality coffee that they didn't know about before.

Plus, let's face it. A diet linked to coffee means the brown java deserves a little extra coverage to whet the appetites.

Please allow just one more round of introductions and backgrounds to three key elements of the 10-Hour Coffee Diet before it's all put together for you in one nice, complete answer. This chapter introduces you to the *3 weird tricks* that are game-changers for you!

Once you understand these three tricks, you will better wrap your arms around the entire 10-Hour Coffee Diet. These three items comprise what I call weird tricks because they, along with intermittent fasting, are the core factors involved in the 10-Hour Coffee Diet's extreme fat loss abilities!

The 10-Hour Coffee Diet's 3 weird tricks that you will use with coffee are:

1. Coconut oil (and *MCT oil*)
2. Grass-Fed Butter (sometimes called *pastured butter*)
3. Protein Powder

Weird Trick #1: Organic Extra Virgin Coconut Oil

I'm not one to throw around the term "miracle" a lot because doing so makes me sound like a snake oil salesman instead of a promoter of healthy products. Still, both from a personal anecdotal experience as well as an intense research of coconut oil for a previous book I wrote, the term "miracle" seems to be within easy grasp given how much coconut oil does for our health.

Oh the benefits of coconut oil!

Here are just a few of them:

- Smaller waistlines
- More energy
- Better-tasting meals
- Healthier hair and skin

In other words, simply adding a healthy coconut oil to your diet, if you change nothing else, *will* begin to aid you in fat loss and should help with better overall well-being.

I will be devoting an entire mini-section to coconut oil later in this book. For now, I want to do a quick rundown of it so you can get right into the 10-Hour Coffee Diet.

Consider these healthy benefits:

- Cleaner and therefore healthier teeth[24]
- Slows and can even reverse Alzheimer's, Parkinson's, and ALS[25]
- Improves Type 1 and Type 2 diabetes[26]
- Improves or heals several skin conditions including fungal infections, acne, eczema, psoriasis, and rosacea[27]
- Kills candida fungus[28]
- Kills many bacteria and viruses
- Can slow, reduce, and even help reverse autism[29]

And it's not just for bodies! For example, here's an easy way to remove stickers from plastics or furniture without resorting to harsh, chemical-laden gunk-removers: mix together equal parts of a little baking soda and coconut oil. Those stickers will come off just about any surface![30]

Coconut oil is one of the most under-utilized ingredients today. Virtually everybody would benefit several ways by adding a good quality coconut oil to their daily lives.

First, a Return to the Notion of Good Fats

To put your weight loss (and health) into high gear, you need to eat more fat. Yes, this does go against much that's been touted for decades.

Fat should comprise as much as 30 to 35% of your diet. The healthy fat you need comes from sources such as healthy oils like coconut and virgin olive oil, organic seeds, and nuts. It's not that fats are good for you; it's that *good* fats are good for you.

There is a huge difference between manufactured fats, bad naturally occurring fats, vegetable oils, soybean oils, and healthy fats.

Unsaturated Fats - The Worst Fats

While sometimes at odds with each other, both the natural health and food experts such as Gary Taubes *and* traditional sources such as the FDA and medical schools agree that trans fats are bad for us. Trans fats *are* bad for us. Trans fats are also called *unsaturated fats*. Stay away from any kind of processed fat or cooking oil labeled trans fat, unsaturated fat, mono-saturated fat, or polyunsaturated fat. This deadly fat messes with your whole body and never in a good way... from your hormones to your heart to your cholesterol.

Polyunsaturated vegetable oils and fats can become toxic and unstable when heated due to the creation of free radicals that damage our cells. Trans fats from hydrogenated oils and margarine are like plastics. They interfere with your cells ability to communicate with each other, which leads to health dysfunction and chaos at the cell level.

The Good Fats

Many fats are great *and required for good health and proper weight levels*. Tropical fats are the best for us. Cook your family's eggs each morning in organic coconut oil, and you can mix it up with extra virgin olive oil too. I use organic coconut oil with eggs every morning (when I eat breakfast). It contains healthy fat and the lauric acid is anti-microbial and fights off bacteria and virus infections.

Organic nuts and seeds are wonderful sources of fats and minerals and vitamins. Make organic nuts and seeds a regular part of your family's diet with a couple of tablespoons of mixed nuts and seeds daily. Did you know that four Brazil nuts each day is all you need to give your body its needed and important selenium? Popping four delicious Brazil nuts is a lot more fun than popping selenium supplements.

We'll get to butter before this chapter is done. But while on the topic of good fats, you've probably heard that margarine is okay, right? Now forget everything you know about it. Margarine is a trans fat. Throw it away *now*. If you just bought a new package of anything labeled, "I can't understand why this delicious yellow stuff isn't butter" then throw it away faster than if it was arsenic in your refrigerator. Please, never use it again.

A lack of natural fats in your diet makes you gain weight. Healthy fats are *essential* for your cells to work properly and eliminate waste and toxins at your cell level... and freeing up your body to lose weight. Fats stabilize blood sugar levels, decrease cravings, and make you feel full. The 10-Hour Coffee Diet would be far less effective if healthy oils were not part of its composition.

Dangers of Low-Fat Mania

In 1982, the American Heart Association, the American Medical Association, and the USDA issued a dire and, unfortunately, very public warning against fat in food. This is why after only a couple of years it seemed as though every product on the supermarket shelves was sold in a "fat free" version. The public's health has degraded ever since as a direct result.

Today some products are difficult to find in a non-fat-free version. Look through the salad dressings in your store to see the large percentage that are fat-free. Walk into any of those Can't-B-Yogurt stores and see how many flavors are fat-free. In some of them, *every flavor* is fat-free. One store I walked into recently had absolutely no yogurts that were sugar-free. And therein lies the problem: to make fat-free "food" good enough for consumers to eat, food makers must add sugar, and loads of it. But the sugar is disguised as High Fructose Corn Syrup, Fructose, Dextrose, maltodextrin, and many other non-sugar-sounding names because if they told the direct truth – that the product is loaded with sugar – you wouldn't buy it even if it also says it is "fat-free."

What's interesting is the result of the four decades that have occurred since that dire warning against fat. The amount of fat in products worldwide has decreased dramatically. According to Dr. Robert H. Lustig[31], M.D., the UCSF Professor of Pediatrics in the Division of Endocrinology, from 1960 to 2000, the percentage of calories from fat has dropped systematically from 45% down to 30%, a move of 1/3rd. While all that fat has been removed from our available foods, the obesity prevalence has increased in that same time period from 14% to 30%, a whopping 200% increase. Less fat in food, but we're far fatter than before.

It's not the fat in foods making us fat. People find, rather quickly, that adding fat back into their diets improves their fat loss ability.

Note: It seems to me that given the current situation – more no-fat and low-fat products line the grocery shelves while we get fatter and fatter as a people – our bodies begin to latch on to any fat we have when it doesn't get a steady supply of fat. This is why adding a healthy fat to our daily regimen, even if we don't change anything else, almost always helps for fat loss.

Sourcing Your Coconut Oil

I know from talking with people who email me for advice that the number one question will be, "What kind of coconut oil should I get?"

The short answer is that you should only get a coconut oil that meets these conditions:

- Is an organic coconut oil
- Is an extra virgin coconut oil

Note: Coconut oil is known as a *saturated fat.* Coconut oil is not prone to oxidation or free radical damage. An unopened jar of virgin coconut oil can last several years, even at room temperature, so feel free to stock up.

An excellent coconut oil is Nutiva's organic extra-virgin coconut oil here: amazon.com/Nutiva-Certified-Organic-Virgin-Coconut/dp/B000GAT6NG

Note: I love the taste of coconuts! If you do, you may be slightly disappointed that most high quality coconut oils don't have a strong coconut flavor. They actually have only a slight buttery flavor for the most part. This buttery flavor and texture makes for a most excellent 10-Hour Coffee Diet coffee, but it doesn't typically add much of a coconut flavor if that is what you're expecting. (Conversely, if you don't care for the taste of coconut, you now know that your extra virgin organic coconut oil won't add that taste you may have been dreading up to this point.)

About MCT and Coconut Oil

MCT is an abbreviation for *Medium Chain Triglycerides.* Coconut oil contains MCTs. You can get MCT oil by itself. If you take coconut oil, you are getting MCT as well. Later you'll see why you may want to try one or the other to see which is best for you, but for now take a moment to learn more about MCT oil.

MCT oil is a fat that works like a carbohydrate in your body. In other words, it provides fuel. Your body is able to utilize MCTs for energy right away and create a thermogenic effect in the process. That is, your body burns more calories than it would without the MCTs. This thermogenic effect means far fewer calories are stored as fat because of the significant number of extra calories burned simply by the mere presence of MCTs.[32]

Dr. Joseph Mercola, M.D., discusses MCTs quite a bit in his research findings. He says:[33]

Coconut oil is also nature's richest source of medium-chain fatty acids (MCFAs), also called medium-chain triglycerides or MCTs. By contrast, most common vegetable or seed oils are comprised of long chain fatty acids (LCFAs), also known as long-chain triglycerides or LCTs.

LCTs are large molecules, so they are difficult for your body to break down and are predominantly stored as fat.

But MCTs, being smaller, are easily digested and immediately burned by your liver for energy -- like carbohydrates, but without the insulin spike. MCTs actually boost your metabolism and help your body use fat for energy, as opposed to storing it, so it can actually help you become leaner.

Note: Dr. Mercola is telling us that the type of fat in coconut oil is extremely difficult for our bodies to store as fat and extremely simple for our bodies to use for fuel. Athletes are learning quickly that coconut oil in their pre- and post-training diets enables them to go further and longer with training than they otherwise could.

Back in the 1940s, farmers discovered this effect accidentally when they tried using inexpensive coconut oil to fatten their livestock.

It didn't work!

Instead, coconut oil made the animals lean, active and satisfied.

Coconut oil has actually been shown to help optimize body weight, which can dramatically reduce your risk of developing Type 2 diabetes. Besides weight loss, boosting your metabolic rate will improve your energy, accelerate healing, and improve your overall immune function.

Coconut oil and MCT oil are metabolism-raisers on overdrive. Such oil's medium-chain triglycerides (MCTs) boost your metabolism and help your body use fat for energy, as opposed to storing it, so it can actually help you become leaner.

Do You Choose Coconut Oil Over MCT or Vice-Versa?

MCT oil is more of a pure form of MCTs than coconut oil. You get a larger concentration of MCTs in MCT oil.

You can find *NOW Foods* MCT oil here: amazon.com/NOW-Foods-100%25-32-Fluid-Ounces/dp/B0019LRY8A

In spite of its richer concentration of MCTs, I recommend that you stick with a high quality coconut oil. Doing so gives you more than enough MCTs and coconut oil is more versatile. In its natural organic form, pure coconut oil is a food meant to be eaten, cooked with, and so on while pure MCT oil is strictly a supplement and not as versatile.

In addition, some might find that MCT oil can cause a little cramping, but any time one begins ingesting more fats, even good fats, initial digestion problems can arise. If you find that you'd like a little digestive help with all the extra fats, consider getting some NOW Super Enzymes and take one with each 10-Hour Coffee Diet coffee. These enzymes prime your system to better digest the fat.

You can get the NOW Super Enzymes on Amazon here: amazon.com/NOW-Foods-Super-Enzymes-Tablets/dp/B0013OXKJA

One advantage that MCT oil brings to the 10-Hour Coffee Diet is its ability to dissolve far easier in coffee. Whether your coffee is hot or cold, MCT oil goes right in and remains in a liquid form that you can easily blend in to the diet's coffee recipe, which you'll learn about shortly. Coconut oil on the other hand is solid until it reaches about room temperature (76 degrees). What this means is that if you drink your coffee lukewarm or cold, coconut oil isn't going to dissolve or mix in as well as it will when the coffee is hot. You'll have to add coconut oil to your coffee recipe when the coffee is still warm unless you don't mind the coconut oil solids (soft solids) in the drink.

In spite of the solid state of coconut oil in any lukewarm or cold drink, it's best for almost everybody reading this book to stick with the tried and true and extremely health-inducing coconut oil. Just be sure to get a pure, organic coconut oil as mentioned previously.

Weird Trick #2: Grass-fed Butter

The second idea (trick) that may be new to many readers is "grass-fed butter."

First of all, you saw earlier how bad margarine is, due to the trans fats that comprise it. One stick of margarine contains a whopping 3 grams of trans fat. Not all calories are the same. More accurately, not all calories affect your body the same. As said above, the MCT oil in coconut oil turns into energy and doesn't store well as fat on our hips. But the trans fats in margarine are as far from the MCTs in coconut oil as it is from butter.

Butter was marginalized (by margarine!) in the 1970s with warnings of its fat, but there is overwhelming research that topples that myth. Butter is better, but there's a butter that's even better than that… grass-fed butter. And, it's probably one of the healthiest foods that you never hear about.

Obviously butter isn't fed grass! Grass-fed butter is butter made from milk from cows that were allowed to eat grass in pastures. Other than some cold winter days here and there, cows should not be fed grains because they were made to eat grass. Most of the milk consumed today is from cows that stand, cradle-to-grave, in one place, pumped full of antibiotics to keep them alive in those conditions, and fed corn and soy grains their entire lives. The resulting milk is inferior and the antibiotics that pass through their systems do us no good at all.

When cows are happy, we're happy. Pasture-raised, grass-fed cows produce the healthiest milk, and if your butter is made from grass-fed cows you have the best indicator that the butter will be as healthy as possible.

> **Note:** When it comes to milk, eggs, chicken, pork, and beef, you should not be as strict about pure "organic" as you should be for other foods such as vegetables, coffee, tea, berries, and the nuts and seeds. The cradle-to-grave antibiotics are bad for the animals and ultimately us, but once in a while we get sick and need an antibiotic and it's perfectly fine if a grass-fed cow that comes down with an infection gets a short-term antibiotic to get well again. By being strictly organic, sick animals cannot be given antibiotics at any time for any reason. This means far more death of the animals and your prices rise accordingly. As long as the meat you eat is grass-fed, locally if at all possible, you are getting about the best possible meat (and eggs and milk) you can.

If your state or locale allows you to buy raw milk from a dairy, and the cows there are grass-fed, you should consider making your own butter. It's simple to make and the raw milk is far better for you than milk that's been squeezed and heated through homogenization and pasteurization.[34] If you, or members of your family, are lactose intolerant (allergic to milk), just know that hardly anyone who is lactose intolerant to processed, store-bought milk is allergic to good, wholesome raw milk.

Another bonus while on the subject of milk, always get whole milk for the same reason you want other good fats in your body. Whole milk, especially grass-fed milk, and grass-fed raw milk, if you can locate it, provides an extremely good fat for your body's lubrication and proper functioning along with several proteins and calcium that is great for you.

Store-Bought Grass-Fed Butter

Let's face it. Most people are busy, far too busy to find a dairy that sells raw milk and go there regularly to buy the milk.

> **Note:** Milk freezes well by the way. So if you do locate a local farm or find a co-op to join where you can get raw milk, feel free to stock up if you have enough freezer space.

Not only do few of us have time to locate and buy raw milk at a dairy, we certainly don't have time to make our own butter at home!

Fortunately, there are good alternatives. You'll need one of these alternatives because grass-fed butter is one key ingredient to the 10-Hour Coffee Diet coffee. It's difficult to get something like butter from Amazon or anywhere else online. Your local Whole Foods (or equivalent upscale or healthy grocery store) should have Kerrygold butter.

At the time of this writing, Kerrygold grass-fed butter is available at Whole Foods for only $2.99 for 8 ounces.

> **Note:** If you don't have Whole Foods, Sprouts, or other health-conscious grocery stores nearby, your local grocer can order Kerrygold grass-fed butter. Tell the manager that you want some and if you can order a case, he's more likely to place the order and more likely to give you a price break over the single-package price. Be sure to ask about a case discount when you ask the manager to order Kerrygold for you.
>
> Kerrygold is available on Amazon, but due to it's extremely high shipping cost it's just not worth buying.

Here's the link to it on Amazon: amazon.com/Kerrygold-Pure-Irish-Butter-Unsalted/dp/B001LNPHNA/

As much as I love Kerrygold, I still want you to consider making your own if you can locate any raw, whole milk in your area. Kerrygold is great, but not perfect. You can come much closer to butter perfection in your own kitchen.

Note: You can leave real butter made from raw milk on your counter without refrigeration. This keeps your butter soft and easy to spread. Eventually, as in months later, homemade butter from raw milk – the way your great grandmother always made it and all grandmothers before her – will get old and sour, but it will *not* go rancid. The sour butter actually isn't bad for you because it has some good lactose fermentation qualities, but really, you can find much better tasting fermented foods such as kefir and homemade yogurt. Still, my primary point is that the butter you buy at the store will go rancid and get old quickly if you don't keep it in your fridge. It's the nature of high-healthy foods, such as raw milk, grass-fed butter... they don't go bad even though they will sour over time.

Still want convincing? Grass-fed and especially organic grass-fed butter is said to provide all of these health benefits:[35]

- Vitamins A, D, E, and K2 (the last three are said to be lacking in today's modern diets)
- Healthful short- and medium-chain fats which support your immune functioning, boost metabolism, and have an anti-microbial property
- Glycospingolipids, a special set of good fatty acids that protect you against gastrointestinal infections, especially the young and elderly
- Trace minerals including zinc, copper, selenium, and iodine
- CLA, or *Conjugated Linoleic Acid,* a substance that provides excellent protection against cancer and that also is a muscle booster in your body
- *Wulzen Factor*, a hormone-like substance that helps prevent joint and muscle stiffness and that enables calcium to more easily be absorbed by your bones rather than your tissues and joints.

Note: The Wulzen Factor is present in butter and cream, but it's destroyed by pasteurization.

If you like the taste of natural and organic ghee (a clarified butter with the milk solids removed), it provides all the health benefits of grass-fed butter.[36] Feel free to substitute ghee for butter in any of your 10-Hour Coffee Diet coffees.

Always get unsalted grass-fed butter. Real salt, such as sea salt, is not bad for you (with the exception of some severe heart patients). You can always add sea salt to any food you use the unsalted grass-fed butter with. As to using grass-fed butter in coffee, however, for taste reasons you'll always want to use unsalted grass-fed butter. So when buying it, choose the unsalted version.

Finally, if the thought of putting butter (or ghee) in your coffee just sounds bad, consider a couple of things before you throw in the towel. If cream in coffee is okay with you, then consider that cream is basically just the fat from whole milk. So is grass-fed butter. Grass-fed butter is a delicious, creamy delight and helps smooth the taste of even the most acidic or bitter coffee (such as the coffee you drink if you buy it pre-ground in a bag from the grocery store shelf).

Weird Trick #3: Protein Powder

The final item you need is a high-quality protein powder. The protein assures no muscle loss will occur as a result of the intermittent fasting protocols used with the diet (remember: if you lose muscle, you slow your metabolism.[37]

Actually, you may find that your lean muscle mass increases with the 10-Hour Coffee Diet when combined with a proper exercise program (especially for those that lift weights).

There are a lot of protein powders on the market. For most people, a whey protein powder is the ideal choice. However, you can use any kind of protein powder except soy!

I usually use ON Gold Standard 100% Whey protein powder. Research conclusively shows that whey protein is superior to any other protein powder you might get.[38] If you don't already have a preferred protein powder, try the ON powder first. The taste is good (chocolate and about 15 other flavors are available) and it goes well in the coffee you'll make for the 10-Hour Coffee Diet coffees.

You can order ON's protein powder here: amazon.com/Optimum-Nutrition-Standard-Double-Chocolate/dp/B000QSNYGI/

Note: As I mentioned before, if you're in the UK you can probably find most or all of these products listed in the Amazon.co.uk website. If you're not in the USA or UK, check your national Amazon website (if you have one) or you can search online or go to a local health food store. Unfortunately, prices vary around the world on products from country to country even after taking exchange rates into consideration. So, you'll have to adjust my later price calculations for the cost of the 10-Hour Coffee Diet as needed.

4
MAKING THE 10-HOUR COFFEE DIET'S COFFEE

If you don't prepare your 10-Hour Coffee Diet's coffee properly, it won't provide the needed nutrition you require to lose fat, feel full, lose sugar and starchy carbohydrate cravings, and to be healthier.

Introducing the 10-Hour Coffee Diet's Coffee

The 10-Hour Coffee Diet is extra-powerful due to several key factors:

1. The addition of protein powder to preserve and protect your muscles
2. Grass-fed butter
3. Organic extra virgin coconut oil
4. Organic, higher quality coffee
5. The unique and most special timing of the 10-Hour Coffee Diet.

In this chapter you will learn the recipe for the 10-Hour Coffee Diet's coffee. A quick review of the fundamental ingredient – coffee – will help solidify some concepts you read in the first chapter:

- Store-bought organic coffee in a larger bag or container is fine. If you want to improve upon the taste, the fresher the coffee you can get, the better it should taste. But the cost will be higher.
- Organic coffee is important given the massive use of pesticides at most coffee plantations around the world (more so than most other foods).
- If you get a coffee bean grinder and begin buying fresh coffee beans, if you grind those beans right before each cup or pot of coffee you make, you'll be blown away by the flavor. But for busy people, this isn't always possible or wanted.

- For those who really want to live on the edge, if your town has one or more specialty coffee shops, your coffee will almost certainly taste exceptional if you buy your beans there. If they roast their own coffee beans locally, you will experience perhaps the most flavorful coffee you will ever drink if you use their beans and ask them some preferred brewing methods they suggest works best for their beans.

What You'll Need To Begin Now

To begin, you're going to need the following:

1. A coffee maker (with coffee of course)
2. A blender
3. Filtered water

Your Coffee Maker

Earlier I discussed ways of making coffee. If you're already a coffee drinker, you no doubt have your own maker already. If you're comfortable with that method, keep using it. At the same time keep the coffee-improvement tips in mind that I've shared with you, such as those reviewed in the previous section. If coffee is going to be a major part of your fat-loss program, and it should be when you begin seeing its results, why not go the extra mile to get amazing tasting coffee as well?

Still, if you are used to store-bought, non-organic, pre-ground, major company blend coffee and you like it and you don't want to change, there's little I can do or should do to convince you otherwise.

Note: Your body will not respond quite as effectively with conventional, non-organic coffee as it can do with organic. If you go against my advice and use regular coffee for this diet, don't blame the diet if you don't get the results you seek.

I discussed the amazing little Aerobie coffee maker in the first chapter. If, instead, you need to get a coffee maker but don't want to go such an unconventional route, for under $20 you can get a personal coffeemaker that's simple to use.

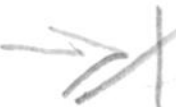

It's the Black & Decker Brew 'n Go Personal Coffee Maker with Travel Mug:

Amazon sells it here: amazon.com/Black-Decker-DCM18S-Personal-Coffeemaker/dp/B00005MF9C

This is one of the most convenient ways to make traditional coffee when convenience is of major importance. Unless you proudly consider yourself one of those self-proclaimed coffee snobs discussed earlier, convenience trumps high quality and this maker is convenient. It isn't perfect. I'm never thrilled to see hot liquids or food in plastic due to the problems with toxins in such plastic leaking into its contents. Also, it's a single-cup brew method so if you are on the 10-Hour Coffee Diet with your spouse then you'll want a coffee maker that makes a larger amount. Still, that single cup size is about the perfect size for each of your coffees on the 10-Hour Coffee Diet so for individuals on the plan, it's not a bad way to go for that reason.

By the way, it makes 15-ounce cups of coffee. If you decide on this handy little coffee maker, factor in this slightly larger-than-normal cup size.

I'm often asked about the K-Cups and Nespresso cups and the similar makers where you have coffee in pre-ground pods, then drop the pod into the maker, and out comes a cup of coffee. These are probably the ultimate in convenience. But that convenience comes with a price and those coffee pods are extremely high priced compared to any other form of coffee. Plus, most of the pods are either aluminum or plastic, two substances you don't want to store hot liquids in that are going to go into your body. But as before, if you already have that and enjoy its coffee, my hat's off to you continuing to use it as you get into the 10-Hour Coffee Diet. But consider moving to a different coffee method and higher quality of coffee when you get the chance.

So from this point forward, I'll assume you have a coffee maker and coffee.

The Blender

The 10-Hour Coffee Diet basically requires a blender.

I say "basically" because you may be able to do all the stirring by hand and you may be able to use a shaker bottle instead of a blender but several aspects of the plan are made *so* much easier having a blender present. The convenience of having a blender actually contributes to many staying on the plan.

If you have a blender, go ahead and use it of course. Even the powerful, upscale industrial-grade blenders such as the Vita-Mix handle the 10-Hour Coffee Diet well, but so do much cheaper blenders. You don't have to spend a lot to get a simple, effective blender. If you don't already have a blender, consider getting the Hamilton Beach Multi-Function 58148A Blender.

You can grab one of these low-cost, but great-functioning, blenders on Amazon here: amazon.com/Hamilton-Beach-58148A-Multi-Function-Blender/dp/B00EI7DPI0/

> **Note:** A huge advantage of this blender for the 10-Hour Coffee Diet is that it holds 40 ounces. Some of the variations of the 10-Hour Coffee Diet will need that extra room due to froth. In addition, the container is glass, meaning that no plastic toxins will be leached into your food, especially from the hot coffee that you will pour into it.

Clean Filtered Water

I suspect that the one element of the 10-Hour Coffee Diet people cheat on the most is water. They cheat by using tap water instead of filtered or bottled water.

In spite of all I've told you about how to source quality coffee, and in spite of the time I took to tell you about the high quality coconut oil and superb whey protein powder, if you get the cheapest of all those ingredients I'd be happier than if you used tap water. The water is the one thing you strongly should consider changing if you're drinking tap water on a consistent basis.

Our bodies are comprised mostly of water. You might have heard the saying, "You are what you eat," but I like to point out that's not accurate. In reality, you are what you *ate* and you also are what you *drank* in the past. Your body, made mostly of water, gets that water primarily from the water you drink and from the water in other drinks you put into your body. If you're stranded, you can go without food for many days, but you will die without water very quickly. If water is what your body needs most to survive and if water is what your body is mostly made from, why would you ever want to put anything but the purest of water in your mouth?

It really makes sense to begin with water if you are going to improve any aspect of your health.

American tap water contains chlorine and other chemicals your municipal water department uses to kill the water's bacteria and other contaminants. But replacing bad contaminants with other bad contaminants doesn't make sense.

> **Note:** Many municipalities in Europe have outlawed the use of chemicals to treat water. They pump oxygen into their water systems. Oxygen will kill bacteria quickly and effectively without putting new contaminants into the water.[39]

Purifying water isn't always easy. Let's face it... turning on your tap is the simplest way to get water. And I've learned not to be too demanding in my writing. Instead of demanding I'll beg you to re-consider using tap water for the water you drink. I want the water you use, whether it's water to make the 10-Hour Coffee Diet's coffee or not, to be pure, clean water. Your body won't have to work nearly as hard dealing with the chemicals in water you drink and can instead route those resources to losing fat and staying healthy. Your cells want the purest water possible and you should consider giving it to them.

Many ways exist, from a full-house reverse osmosis water treatment system to small filtered pitchers. Whatever you do, using something to decrease the long-term effects of all those chemicals can only help you. Plus your coffee will always taste better!

Buying bottled water isn't always convenient (or healthy) and it certainly gets expensive. A much cheaper option, at least to get you started, is the simple Brita Slim Water filter.

Right now on Amazon, this Brita is *under $10* and that includes the filter! Here it is: amazon.com/Brita-Slim-Water-Filter-Pitcher/dp/B0000AP7NV

Note: As an added health bonus, this Brita filter is BPA-free. This means its plastic toxins will not leach into your water as it does its job.

The Recipe – Making Your 10-Hour Coffee Diet's Coffee

Finally, the section you've been waiting for! I suspect you'll appreciate the information that came before, however. Trying to cover details about coconut oil right in the middle of the 10-Hour Coffee Diet's recipe would confuse things greatly.

Note: I'll be discussing possible modifications to the original coffee recipe as we go forward. Starting in the next chapter, I'll introduce the timeline that you follow (hint: it's a 10-Hour timeline!) as well as give you alternative timelines after that. The original coffee and the first timeline are easiest and if you can stick with those, great. But we all differ in our tastes and our schedules and lifestyle. It's nice to have options. I'll try to keep everything simple and make it easy for you to decide which one you want to pick and use. And it's always fine to mix it up and see if one recipe or schedule is better for you than another.

Please keep in mind, the coffee itself is just one important aspect of the 10-Hour Coffee Diet. It is certainly not the whole diet. The timing of when you have the coffee and how many you drink each day is vital to learn. That "protocol" of the diet – the timing and amounts – begins in the next chapter and shows you exactly how to perform the intermittent fast discussed earlier.

For the traditional 10-Hour Coffee Diet Plan's coffee, here is all you do:

1. Make 12 to 15 ounces of coffee. This is straight drip or brewed coffee. If you prefer espresso, you don't want to make 12 ounces of espresso! For espresso lovers, go ahead and make 4 ounces of espresso and add enough hot water to get to 12 ounces of coffee. (This is one way to make the coffee traditionally known as an *Americano*.)
2. Pour the coffee into your blender.
3. Put 1 to 1.5 tablespoons of coconut oil or MCT oil, depending on which you want to use, into the blender's coffee while the coffee is still hot. Adding the coconut oil to the hot coffee liquefies the coconut oil from its previously solid state. (MCT oil is a liquid at room temperature already, so it doesn't matter.)

Note: If you are prone to stomach problems, or are using MCT oil for the first time, use only one tablespoon. This will help get your stomach used to the MCT oil. The NOW Super Enzymes help your fat digestion, as mentioned earlier, if you need a little extra help when you first begin the coconut oil or MCT oil.

4. Add 1 to 1.5 tablespoons of grass-fed butter to the blender. The coffee will still be warm enough to melt the butter. Even if the butter is cold and doesn't fully melt immediately, the blending action will be enough to blend the butter into the coffee.

Note: If you eat a lot of good fats, such as organic seeds and nuts, use organic extra virgin olive oil on salads, and cook with coconut oil, then you only need to use a single tablespoon in each 10-Hour Coffee Diet coffee. If you don't regularly get a lot of good fats, consider using 1.5 tablespoons.

5. Add approximately 20 grams of your protein powder to the blender's solution.
6. Turn the blender on low-to-medium speed. In about 10 seconds, the mixture will look smooth and should be ready to drink.

You've Made the Coffee but Whatever You Do Don't Drink It!

Actually, you can *begin* drinking it now but your goal is to sip the 10-Hour Coffee over a period of 10 to 20

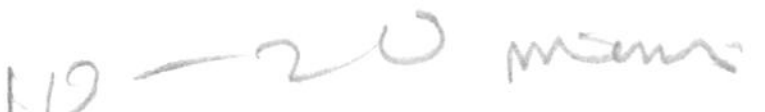

minutes. This gives your body a good time-range to absorb the nutrients in the coffee's fats and to give the coffee a chance to permeate your cells and boost your metabolism.

The double-blast of good, healthy, waistline-reducing fats, along with the boosted metabolism is going to super-charge your fat loss!

But there's one more piece to the puzzle: The daily diet plan that includes the coffee above. We'll discuss how to lay out your days in the next chapter.

> **Note:** I don't care for hot drinks. If you want to add an ice cube or two, it will weaken the 10-Hour Coffee Diet's coffee, but won't weaken its effectiveness. Below, you'll learn another way to cool the drink without using ice.

2 Optional Items Can Accent Your Coffee

As good as the 10-Hour Coffee Diet's coffee is, especially if you go with a specialty or even a medium quality coffee, some people want or need just a little extra flavor and sweetness.

Stevia for Sweetness

Feel free to add Stevia as needed for a nice sweet accent to your coffee's flavor.

Stevia comes from the Stevia plant and when you buy the right kind, 100% of the Stevia sweetener is real and natural. Stevia doesn't raise your blood sugar levels and has a zero-carb impact on your body's fat.

Stevia comes in packets or a smaller shaker. Both are easy to carry with you. Whatever you do, be careful that the Stevia you get is made in America where controls are strict and it's always best to get a brand that doesn't add fillers and hidden negative ingredients such as alcohol, dextrose (a form of sugar), maltodextrin (a high glycemic filler used to prevent clumping), or inulin (a hard to digest fiber that acts as a filler). Those fillers simply lower your cost at the detriment of true Stevia's inert nature. From a taste perspective, Stevias loaded with fillers also require that you to use far more to get a good taste.

My ready-to-go Stevia used to be Kal. Unfortunately, they moved the extraction process to China and the quality has taken a big step backwards. I tried out Better Stevia packets along with Nustevia packets and even though Kal is a lot less potent compared to before, I still have to rate it above those two. At this point I can't give a strong recommendation, but here is a link the Kal Stevia on Amazon: amazon.com/Kal-Pure-Stevia-Extract-Powder/dp/B000VRSR84

The Addition of Almond Milk

Another item to consider as you enter the exciting world of the 10-Hour Coffee Diet is unsweetened almond milk. Most grocery stores carry some form of almond milk. It may go by names such as *Almond Breeze* or *Silky Almond.* It usually costs less than $3 for a half gallon.

> **Note:** Although I think the addition of real, organic vanilla to coffee and some other items can accent the flavor and may provide additional health benefits, do *not* get vanilla-flavored almond milk. Always get the "regular" or "plain" flavor and make sure it says 'unsweetened' on the container. The addition of vanilla flavoring, even in the organic almond milks, often adds a faux vanilla extract whose effects, are not well known yet. If you want a vanilla-flavored almond milk, get a high quality organic vanilla extract and add a drop or two to your almond milk instead of getting vanilla-flavored milk.

For your 10-Hour Coffee Diet coffee, you can add 4 to 8 ounces of almond milk. It's only 15-30 calories (if you were wondering).

The 10-Hour Coffee Diet Recipe Using Almond Milk and Optionally Stevia

Almond milk has been such a favorite add-on to the 10-Hour Coffee Diet that I need to give you a modified way of making your coffee if you decide to use almond milk.

> **Note:** You can add Stevia any time during the making of your 10-Hour Coffee Diet's coffee. You can wait until right before you drink it to add the sweetener or add it before blending process. Adding Stevia before blending your coffee drink will help mix the Stevia far better than adding it after to pour the

coffee into your cup to drink it.

The last thing I want to do is confuse you with a lot of options, yet I must give alternatives both to the coffee recipe as well as the timing of when you drink your coffee. Lifestyles and tastes are too different to give a one-stop-fits-all answer. So know this: If you've made the traditional coffee described earlier in this chapter and want to try almond milk and possibly Stevia, then instead of following the previous steps, follow the ones below. To put it more simply, if you don't use almond milk ignore this alternative recipe.

Keep in mind the almond milk is going to cool the coffee down. Even if you use very cold almond milk, the fresh-brewed coffee's heat will keep the almond milk from making the drink extremely cold. But it will be closer to lukewarm than cold. You can add an ice cube or two to make it colder or you can drink it lukewarm.

For the traditional 10-Hour Coffee Diet Plan's coffee WITH almond milk, here is all you do:

1. Make 12 to 15 ounces of coffee. This is straight drip or brewed coffee. If you prefer espresso, you don't want to make 12 ounces of espresso! For espresso lovers, go ahead and make 4 ounces of espresso and add enough hot water to get to 12 ounces of coffee. (This is one way to make the coffee traditionally known as an *Americano.*)
2. Do *not* pour the coffee into your blender yet. While the coffee is brewing, put 4 to 8 ounces of almond milk into the blender.
3. Add 20 grams of protein powder to the blender.
4. Add the hot coffee to the blender.
5. Immediately put 1 to 1.5 tablespoons of coconut oil or MCT oil, depending on which you want to use, onto the blender's coffee while the coffee is still hot. Adding the coconut oil to the hot coffee, as opposed to adding it at the bottom where the cold almond milk resides, help liquefy the coconut oil from its previously solid state. (MCT oil is a liquid at room temperature already so it doesn't matter when you add it.)
6. Immediately add 1 to 1.5 tablespoons of grass-fed butter on top of the hot coffee in the blender. The coffee will still be warm enough to melt the butter during the blending process.
7. Turn the blender on low-to-medium speed. In about 10 seconds, the mixture will look smooth and should be ready to drink.

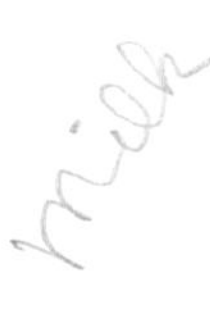

Note: Feel free to use almond milk to accent your coffee like a cream instead of using the full 4 to 8 ounces. Although you *can* use regular whole milk, the lactose sugar means you should limit it to 2 ounces maximum. Some people like whole whipping cream, but for that you need to limit it to only 1 ounce. Don't do both milk or cream and almond milk. And you don't need the almond milk or anything else! Many people love the taste of the 10-Hour Coffee Diet's coffee with just the butter, protein powder, and coconut oil alone. The almond milk can be an added bonus to give it a milky taste by just putting a spoonful or two into your coffee. So you don't need to use the full amount of almond milk mentioned.

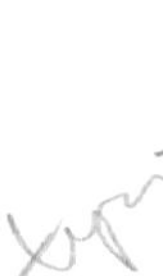

If you do happen to use regular milk as a 1- or 2-ounce creamer in your coffee, never use skim milk. Dairy farmers feed calves skim milk to *fatten them up!* As illogical as it may seem at first, it's worth mentioning once more than good fat allows your body to let go of excess stored fat. The extra calories that whole milk brings are good fat calories, just as the fat in coconut oil and grass-fed butter is good.

If You Want Cold Coffee

If you like your drinks cold, it's fine to drink the 10-Hour Coffee Diet's coffee cold. Although you could keep adding ice after you make the 10-Hour Coffee Diet coffee, doing that weakens the taste as mentioned earlier.

A better way is to brew coffee ahead of time and chill it by storing the coffee in a glass pitcher in your refrigerator. Unlike coffee that gets old quickly after brewing, if you refrigerate coffee, the freshness is much slower to leave the drink than it is at room temperature.

The recipe is the same as above, the traditional method or the method using almond milk, except you obviously don't brew coffee right before you make the diet drink. But keep in mind the butter, and especially the coconut oil, may not liquefy as fully as they would as compared to fresh-brewed, hot coffee.

This has never once been a problem for me. I sometimes get a sort of smooth little bit of coconut oil that hasn't liquefied in the blender. The cold coffee makes it even harder for the coconut oil to liquefy so the coconut oil fights the cold by staying as solid as possible. This is the only trade-off I've found; the bits of coconut oil solids. In addition, the effectiveness of the butter and coconut oil are not reduced by any amount even if they haven't fully melted by the time you drink the coffee.

What about Soy Milk?

Please stay away from soy milk!

Soy puts excess estrogen into our bodies. For females, food shouldn't be increasing our estrogen... and for the men, estrogen certainly shouldn't be coming from food. There are enough estrogen-producing *parabens* in the environment and our plastic food containers to load us up with plenty of estrogen and we don't need more from a food source like soy milk that is easily substituted with the likes of almond milk or healthy, whole, raw, cow's milk.[40] I'll discuss more about these problems later.

There is controversy over soy as to whether or not it's as harmful as some of us suspect from the research we've read thoroughly.[41] Still, with the massive and growing body of evidence that soy has not been the health food it was made out to be, why risk your family's health by adding it to their diets?

Note: Soy sauce is a fermented soy product and does not have the side effects that soy is now said to produce.

5
THE PROTOCOLS – WHEN YOU DRINK THE 10-HOUR COFFEE DIET'S COFFEE

Now that you've seen the recipe, understand the benefits to modified fasting, and realize how crucial good fats are to your fat loss, the final piece of the puzzle can be given: *when* you drink the coffee.

This chapter explains the exact timing of the 10-Hour Coffee Diet. All the elements come together here and you'll finally see the details of the intermittent fasting that you'll be doing along the way.

The Traditional 10-Hour Coffee Diet's Daily Protocol (Coffee-Coffee-Dinner)

Here is the primary schedule for drinking your 10-Hour Coffee Diet's coffee and for eating your meals. If you can maintain this schedule you can expect fantastic results. The combination of the coffee, the good fats, the intermittent fasting, and the protein powder work in an amazing combination to drop fat and maintain and lean muscle mass.

Throw in some exercise and you'll shred the fat and your body's metabolism will go into overdrive.

If some, or all, of this schedule won't work for you, this chapter finishes with several alternatives that can work for you. Be sure to try the first schedule, or protocol, first because it's the best one to follow for daily long-term use. Before this chapter ends you'll have plenty of options to choose from. If you find that some weeks, perhaps due to travel or holidays, you must adjust, feel free to move from the traditional plan to an alternative plan and back again as needed.

Do This For Six Days a Week

Following the traditional plan, for six days a week you will do the 10-Hour Coffee Diet schedule presented below. It's a 10-Hour plan in that about ten hours pass from when you awaken to when you eat dinner. It is during those hours that you drink the coffee. This combines with, what is in reality, a modified 24-hour fast (it won't seem like that long of a fast due to the coffee and its additives that comprise the 3 weird tricks and because part of the time is when you are sleeping). While on the plan six days a week, you only eat primarily for dinner and almost 24 hours will go by between dinners.

Note: It's the 10-Hour Coffee Diet coffee that actually keeps this diet on the level of a simple intermittent fast instead of a 24-hour fast. In one respect, you get the extra advantages of a 24-hour fast with the ease of being able to follow an intermittent fast due to the nutrients and coffees during the day.

It may seem that drinking only the coffee during the first ten hours of your day causes you to be hungry. Almost nobody finds that to be a problem, especially after the first day or two. Later we'll address how to handle hunger that possibly appears once in a while.

1. Upon waking up (or up to an hour after waking), make your 10-Hour Coffee Diet's coffee (see previous chapter) and drink it over a period of 10 to 20 minutes.
2. At your normal lunchtime, drink another 10-Hour Coffee Diet coffee.
3. At your usual dinnertime, eat dinner.

It is simple because simple is one of the most effective ways to continue your long-term compliance to the plan.

Here is a sample outline of the spacing of the 10-Hour Coffee coffees and your dinner. Note that the exact times are unimportant, as you'll adjust them to fit your schedule:

1. You wake up at 7:30 am.
2. You have your first 10-Hour Coffee Diet coffee with additives at 8:00 am.
3. Drink your second 10-Hour Coffee Diet coffee anywhere between 12 and 1 pm.
4. You eat dinner approximately at 6:00 pm.

Those are the key points of the diet along with the timing you will shoot for. Although your schedule will probably make you have to modify the suggested times I gave above, it's important to maintain the 10-hour time frame (8 to 6 is a total of 10 hours). If you go longer before eating your nighttime meal, you risk losing the powerful muscle mass protection the two earlier coffees gave you with the fats and especially with the protein powder. (Remember, maintaining or increasing your lean muscle maintains or speeds up your metabolism, thus speeding up fat loss. Losing muscle slows down your metabolism and fat loss.)

Note: Drink as much water as you want any time, morning or afternoon or night. Water helps suppress your appetite and the coffee is a mild diuretic so you'll want to replenish fluids throughout the day. Never get thirsty; drink water regularly. Just be sure not to drink a lot of water within 30 minutes before or after each of the two 10-Hour Coffee Diet coffees. You want the coffee to have maximum effect and not be diluted by too much water in your stomach at the same time. Any plain tea is also fine any time during the day.

About Your Dinner

Your dinner's requirements are simple: Eat a *sensible* dinner. You'll get better results if you eat a healthy dinner, but you'll still lose weight if you eat a dinner that isn't quite so healthy. It's okay to enjoy some of your favorite foods.

If you can eat a dinner of grass-fed beef or free-range poultry, or wild Alaskan salmon, along with plenty of non-starchy, colorful vegetables, you can eat as much as you want. Eat until you're full (not stuffed), even if it means extra helpings.

The glycemic impact of such a meal won't set you back one bit from the work you did earlier in the day with your coffees.

Note: I repeat that you can eat *anything you* want for dinner and still lose fat. To the extent that you eat breads and pasta and dessert for dinner, as opposed to non-starchy, colorful vegetables and good meat, you will not lose the fat quite as effectively. Each night your body will somewhat reset if you feed it a lot of carbohydrates and you'll backtrack a step even though the next day's pre-dinner 10-Hour Coffee Diet's coffees should put you ahead two steps.

Fortunately, most people find they don't want starches or desserts at dinner. This is directly due to the coconut oil's property of suppressing what your body would otherwise crave without that healthy fat in your system.

What About Fruit?

I haven't mentioned fruit. From this point forward, I'd rather you treat fruit like a dessert. It's something nice to have, certainly better than donuts if you want something sweet, but limit your intake to limit the glycemic impact on your body. If you love fruit, you'll want to have a piece for dinner. That's fine. Berries are probably the best choice for fruits due to all the antioxidants they're loaded with.

Note: Whatever you do, if you want fruit eat the actual fruit such as an apple with its skin. Do not drink fruit juice. The lack of fiber sends that fruit's sugar – *fructose* – straight into your system where it tends to store as fat.

If You Get Hungry Before You Eat

People who eat high carbohydrate breakfasts for a long time before moving to the 10-Hour Coffee Diet are most at risk of getting hungry late morning even with the delicious and nutritious coffee they drink after waking. This will pass! The reason you are craving food is due to habit as well as your body's natural tendency to crave more and more carbohydrates, the more carbohydrates you feed it.

Your body wants to adjust out of this endless carb loading. The protein powder will give you long-term energy and the fats give you short-term energy, as well as the caffeine in the coffee itself. If you feel you want to eat even though you have plenty of energy, you *know* that the hunger is not real. Your body is not telling you it needs nutrients or fuel. The carbs still left in your body and the habitual eating of early-morning carbs are the only reasons you think you're hungry. By the second or third day, it will seem like a miracle because your body wants to get off the roller coaster you're on and the good fats and healthy protein are going to help your body get off the roller coaster quickly.

Consider What Has Now Happened

Perhaps you can now see why I spent so much time before this chapter preparing you for the 10-Hour Coffee Diet. The actual protocol for the traditional diet is extremely simple: 2 "cups" of 10-Hour Coffee Diet coffee and one meal. If I'd led with the schedule, given how deceptively simple it appears, you would no doubt have all sorts of questions about how you could be expected to go the first ten hours of your day without food.

The 10-Hour Coffee Diet's coffee *almost universally* keeps its dieters from feeling hungry at all. More important, the good fats that you put in your system have an added bonus: they tend to eliminate or at the least drastically reduce sugar cravings. If you think you have sugar cravings, you may have a sugar addiction. Today's "sugar" isn't even sugar – today's product used in place of sugar are almost exclusively made from High Fructose Corn Syrup, a substance that is far worse than sugar.[42] Many will find that their sugar cravings are virtually non-existent as early as the first week on the 10-Hour Coffee Diet.

Rest on the Seventh Day

Given that the 10-Hour Coffee Diet is a 6-day diet schedule, feel free to take the seventh day off and eat what you want.

I can't stress the next sentence enough! After six days on the 10-Hour Coffee Diet, even at the end of your first week on it, you're not going to feel any desire to go out and binge on a bunch of cookies, cakes, donuts, and you will almost surely not even want three full meals. Your body's metabolism will already be adjusting to your added boost from the previous days of your new diet. Plus, the good and healthy fats you put into your body those six days act as a super-charging agent to dampen almost all desire to overeat. You should also crave sweets far less than before.

Whatever you do on the seventh day, eat anything and everything you *want* to eat. Just don't eat something because you're free to eat anything. Mentally, you can tell yourself that you haven't had chocolate cake all week so a couple of pieces on the seventh day will be a nice reward. But eat that cake only *if you actually crave the cake!* Don't eat it as a reward for not eating cake all week because you're sort of telling yourself a lie if you do – that cake is no reward, it's a *punishment*! It will reverse some of the good you did in the 10-Hour Coffee Diet you stuck to the previous six days.

So promise yourself right now – on the seventh day you will eat anything and everything you truly *want.*

You Can Still Do the Coffee

Anyone on the 10-Hour Coffee Diet Plan can still use the diet's "loaded up" coffees on the seventh day if they want. If you continue them, switch off the 10-Hour Coffee Diet scheduling. The most important thing is that on the seventh day, I want you to have two to three meals that day.

Why is that you may ask?

I simply don't know what you're eating for the one meal each day of the 10-Hour Coffee Diet. If you repeatedly eat bad foods, or the same thing over and over, you may cause a deficiency in the nutrients you take in. By having a second meal on this seventh day each week, you can bring more variety to your food intake and thus, hopefully, broaden your nutrient intake to alleviate any potential or possible nutrient deficiencies.

I'm not there with you watching how you eat. If you are going to do this diet regularly, and over the long term, then I feel more comfortable advising you to not do a strict 10-Hour Coffee Diet day all seven days a week due to possible nutrient deficiency. This is not to scare you about the diet. You're most likely getting far more nutrients from the 10-Hour Coffee Diet as compared to your normal diet. But be alert so you eat a variety of foods for your meals to help broaden your nutrient intake.

> **Note:** I want chocolate from time to time and maybe you do too. I want to tell you about a chocolate that is good for you! It's chocolate bars made from high-content cacao (that's the pre-cocoa, the bean used to make traditional chocolate), typically found in a dark chocolate form such as the *Ghirardelli Chocolate Intense Dark Midnight Reverie.* You will find that the higher quality dark chocolate bars list the percentage of cacao content. The closer to 100% the cacao content is, the *less the impact that chocolate will have on your belly, thighs, and hips.* (Yes, they do make 100% cacao content bars.) This dark chocolate cacao contains a high amount of fermentation and is very good for your body. High cacao content is much less sweet than a cacao content of only 50% or less. You will find that most chocolates are far too sweet for you after a couple of weeks on your new diet, and you will love the taste of that much healthier chocolate cacao in its natural dark chocolate form.

If You Take Vitamins and Minerals

While on the 10-Hour Coffee Diet, continue to take whatever vitamins and minerals you take now. If you take a liquid vitamin or mineral supplement upon waking up, go ahead and take it and wait an extra half hour to drink your 10-Hour Coffee Diet coffee. If you take supplements in pill form, feel free to take them at your regular times without any impact on the diet.

> **Note:** Some of your supplements may require that you take them with food. Feel free to consider any of your coffees "food." The fat and protein content will do everything necessary to carry those nutrients through your system as intended.

Alternative 10-Hour Coffee Diet Plans

Several factors can keep you from following the traditional 10-Hour Coffee Diet protocol, but it's the most effective long-term version. This is the 10-Hour Coffee Diet protocol you read about above. I would ask that before you try any of the following alternatives that you give the original plan a solid try, at least the first six days, before you change things up and try one of the following alternatives.

Alternative #1: An Extra Coffee (Coffee-Coffee-Coffee-Dinner)

This first alternative helps those who just can't seem to make it to dinner without getting overly hungry. Extremely active people might complain about hunger in the mid-afternoons after their noontime 10-Hour Coffee Diet coffee and before their dinner at about 6 pm.

If this is your problem, try this alternative before you try the others, especially for the first few weeks of your diet. Much of the "hunger" is little more than habit. Your lean muscle loss will be non-existent due to the first two 10-Hour Coffee Diet coffees so your body will not generally crave nutrition before dinner rolls around. Still, it seems to be a problem for some people and the easiest way to stay on track is to add an afternoon 10-Hour Coffee Diet coffee as follows:

1. Upon waking up, make your 10-Hour Coffee Diet's coffee (see previous chapter) and drink it over a period of 10 to 20 minutes.
2. At your normal lunchtime, drink another 10-Hour Coffee Diet coffee.
3. At about 3:30 to 4:30 pm, have a third 10-Hour Coffee Diet coffee. Don't modify the recipe, make the regular amount and add the all-important 3 Weird Tricks (quality whey protein powder, grass-fed butter (or ghee), and coconut oil (or MCT oil).
4. Try to eat dinner a little later than normal to give your body its full opportunity to utilize the nutrients from that third coffee. Eating as late as 7 or 8 pm is fine.

Alternative #2: A Post-Dinner Snack (Coffee-Coffee-Dinner-Snack)

There may be two reasons why you need a small snack within three hours of dinner:

1. You find that you wake up in the middle of the night and don't fall back to sleep for an hour or more. This is typically due to a lack of fat remaining in your system and your body is waking you up in an effort to get you to eat something. The large amount of fats you're taking in the first ten hours of the day should be ample to counter this, but some people may find they still have the problem in the early weeks of the diet.
2. Right before bedtime, or possibly in the middle of the night, you get a craving for munchies. Right before bed, if it's been more than three hours since your dinner, it's too late to eat.

If either happens to you, you should eat a snack within three hours after dinner. A perfect snack would be some organic seeds or nuts. Even better, have some organic almond butter. If you can keep some organic beef jerky in your house, that protein and fat combination makes an excellent pre-bedtime snack and should go a long way towards giving you a healthful, full night's sleep.

To be complete, here is the plan for this alternative protocol:

1. Upon waking up make your 10-Hour Coffee Diet's coffee (see previous chapter) and drink it over a period of 10 to 20 minutes.
2. At your normal lunchtime, drink another 10-Hour Coffee Diet coffee.
3. At your usual dinnertime, eat dinner.
4. Within three hours of finishing dinner, even if it's right before you go to bed, eat a snack. The more healthy fat the snack has, such as Mary's Gone seed crackers dipped in organic avocado, the better you will sleep and the more satisfied your nightly craving will be.

Note: This alternative's real drawback is that you lose two or three hours of your modified 24-hour fast. Instead of going, effectively, 24 hours between actual meals, you are going only 21 hours. Certainly, it's still quite effective though.

Alternative #3: Swapping Lunch for Dinner (Coffee-Lunch-Coffee)

I strongly advise you to resist this alternative protocol unless you have tried the previous ones for a couple of weeks or more. Earlier in this book, I discussed why the saying "breakfast is your most important meal of the day" is a myth. The later in the day you eat, especially if you perform an intermittent fast and don't eat any actual food for the majority of the day, the better your body processes your food and the better your body can access and absorb the nutrients in the food.

Food exists not to taste good. We need food to live. It's fantastic that a lot of good food tastes good, making life far more enjoyable. But when you eat, your body looks at the food as possible nutrients to take advantage of as much as possible.

In the morning hours, your body still retains a few of its sleeping detox functions. Eating breakfast early in the morning stops that detox because your body must transfer resources to digestion.

Eating lunch instead of dinner turns out to be a less effective – but still an effective – way of losing fat through intermittent fasting. As long as you take proper nutrients outside of your lunch hours, through the good fats and protein in the 10-Hour Coffee Diet coffees, you'll certainly lose fat. But it won't be as effective as waiting until dinner to eat. This is true even if you eat a *larger* dinner than lunch!

Still, if you need the meal in the middle of the day because you aren't getting to dinner easily in spite of the previous alternatives you've tried or you have a business lunch, it's great to go on this alternative for a day whenever you need to. If you must maintain this schedule forever, that is fine, but try to return to a dinnertime meal.

1. Upon waking up, make your 10-Hour Coffee Diet's coffee (see previous chapter) and drink it over a period of 10 to 20 minutes.
2. At your normal lunchtime, skip the regularly scheduled 10-Hour Coffee Diet coffee and instead eat a full meal.
3. About 6 pm, drink your second 10-Hour Coffee Diet coffee of the day.

Although eating earlier will not trigger *quite* the fat loss that eating later will, you are still performing a modified 24-hour fast by going about 24 hours between actual meals.

Note: You *can* add a third helping of the 10-Hour Coffee Diet's coffee with lunch or in the evening hours (8 to 10 pm) depending on your energy levels and what you need to do that night. Most people find they don't need the third one. Plus, the caffeine late at night may affect your sleep. So, pay attention to your sleep patterns if you begin doing this.

You might very well want to switch to this alternative as social situations demand. For example, if you know you're going out to lunch with friends or co-workers, then simply have the coffee in the morning and at dinner that day. Problem solved and you can return to the original 10-Hour Coffee Diet schedule the following day.

Alternative #4: Break Your Fast with Breakfast (Breakfast-Coffee-Coffee)

If you've been reading along all the alternatives so far, you probably suspect I'll do my best to steer you away from making your one meal of the day, six days each week, breakfast. Your body hasn't completed its housekeeping yet, such as all its detoxing. If you really crave food in the mornings, it's most likely due to being in the habit of eating a high-carbohydrate breakfast regularly for years.

If you eat fruit, cereal, store-bought sugary yogurts, pancakes, waffles, toast, and other traditional breakfast food, your body will keep craving those carbs for a while after you begin the 10-Hour Coffee Diet. The reason your body does this is there are no nutrients in that kind of food, other than the fruit.

I suggest you go all out and do your best to maintain one of the previous alternatives.

But you're only human, right? If you and your body demand that your primary meal be breakfast, use this protocol when necessary. Just hop back on to another alternative protocol as quickly as possible. Use this timing protocol sparingly.

Here is the protocol to follow:

1. Upon waking up, eat breakfast. The higher the content of good meat, raw whole milk, vegetables such as tomatoes (actually a tomato is a fruit but mimics the effects of vegetables in our bodies), fermented food such as homemade yogurt or store-bought Greek plain organic yogurt, and the lower the amount of cereals and breads you eat, the longer your energy will last the rest of the day.
2. At noon, make your 10-Hour Coffee Diet's coffee (see previous chapter) and drink it over a period of 10 to 20 minutes.
3. About 6 pm, drink another 10-Hour Coffee Diet coffee.
4. If and only if you need one, you can drink another one between 6 pm and your bedtime. Obviously you need to monitor your sleep patterns and not have caffeine that late if it affects your sleep at all. Studies conclusively show that broken sleep will inhibit your fat loss dramatically.[43]

Note: Feel free to have a 10-Hour Coffee Diet coffee with your breakfast. Those fats and proteins, combined with the metabolic effect of the coffee, will enable you to start your day with energy that should easily last through your next coffee, even if you eat an otherwise sluggish breakfast.

Alternative #5: Eating Two Later Meals (Coffee-Lunch-Coffee-Dinner)

The best choice to complement your dinner meal is lunch. That way you won't break your fast from dinner to lunch (the next day) as early as you would if the second meal is breakfast. In addition, several intermittent fasting programs utilize both the lunch and dinner meals as part of an intermittent fast that is broken only during the hours of noon (lunch) to 8 pm.[44]

Here is the protocol you'll follow:

1. Upon waking, make your 10-Hour Coffee Diet's coffee (see previous chapter) and drink it over a period of 10 to 20 minutes.
2. At 12 pm or later, eat lunch.
3. At about 2-3 pm, drink another 10-Hour Coffee Diet coffee.
4. About 6-7 pm, eat dinner.

Be sure that your lunch and dinner meals are not spaced more than 6 hours apart. This maintains an 18-hour modified fast.

Note: Really, this (and the next) alternative schedule is best for people not as concerned about fat loss, but who want to gain the health, gut, and brain benefits that intermittent fasting provides.

Alternative #6: Eating Two Meals Earlier in the Day (Breakfast-Lunch-Coffee)

Of all the plans, this is the weakest for fat loss. Having said that, you *should lose fat* anyway, just not nearly what you would on one of the other protocols.

Here is this modified plan:

1. Upon waking up, drink one 10-Hour Coffee Diet coffee and eat a meal for breakfast.
2. At 12 pm or later, eat lunch *and* a 10-Hour Coffee Diet coffee.
3. About 6 pm, drink a third 10-Hour Coffee Diet coffee. As always, the recipe for your 10-Hour Coffee Diet coffee never varies, whether you drink it alone or with a meal, although you can reduce the amount of water in the coffee when drinking it with a meal.

If you must have two meals and follow either this or the previous protocol, try your best to eat a reduced meal over what you may be used to before you began the 10-Hour Coffee Diet plan. Your breakfast should be smaller to give your still-wakening body a chance to utilize all its resources for your day.

Alternative #7: Raw/Vegan Food with These Coffees Until Dinner

If you only eat raw vegetables or are a vegan, as long as you eat no starchy carbs, you may supplement your usual pre-dinner coffees with some vegan food such as raw vegetables. It's probably best not to mix in nuts and seeds too much; you don't need their fat due to the fat content in the 10-Hour Coffee Diet's coffee.

Even if you aren't normally a vegan-kind of eater, this alternative protocol provides for fat loss greater than the protocol with two meals. Keep your raw munching on a hit-and-run scale and move on... then later you eat a little of something else.

The 10-Hour Coffee Diet helps repair one of the weaknesses of a typical vegan diet. That is, it provides healthy fats and proteins that aren't always available to the vegan eater. For dinner you can eat anything you want. If you want to maintain a vegan diet, just eat your usual vegan fare. Otherwise, eat whatever you want given the parameters above. If you are a strict vegan, I understand that the 10-Hour Coffee Diet coffees may not be a fit for how you eat. You'll have to decide whether these coffees fit your lifestyle.

Alternative #8: Advanced Fat Loss, A Super-Charged 10-Hour Coffee Diet (Coffee-Coffee-Coffee-Coffee)

One of the most powerful body-changing concepts you can consider is made possible with an ultimate 10-Hour Coffee Diet alternative protocol.

> **Note**: Only follow this alternative protocol one to three days at a time. It is, in effect, a 1- to 3-day modified full fast.

What you do is simple. Drink three to four 10-Hour Coffee Diet coffees each day. You don't eat any food or take in any type of calories other than the calories in the 10-Hour Coffee Diet coffees. So, that also means no kind of liquid calories. Follow this plan from one to three days and no more at a time.

The loss of solid food to digest during this short-term modified fast helps create a mini detox that cleanses your body. That rest from digesting food frees up a tremendous amount of resources for other kinds of housekeeping chores your body needs to do. The lack of food also causes a reduction in calories, obviously helping with weight loss.

When given the chance, your body is very good at going into places where it didn't have time or resources to go into before, at the cellular level, to do some maintenance.

Once you return to another version of the 10-Hour Coffee Diet, please don't return to this advanced fat loss version for a week or more. Never follow it regularly. Use this extreme fat-loss alternative to "wake-up" your fat loss and surprise your body with extra resources.

> **Note:** If you take daily vitamins and minerals, keep taking them. They don't count as food in this case, although they literally are food. If you're on prescribed medicines, certainly don't break their protocol either.

If any of your vitamins, minerals, or medicines requires that you take them with food, be sure to take them right after you drink one of your 10-Hour Coffee Diet coffees. Monitor yourself to make sure you don't feel any stomach upset. If you do, stop this alternative immediately and eat a small meal. The next day, return to the original 10-Hour Coffee Diet Plan or one of the alternatives that work for you.

If any of your vitamins, minerals, or medicines requires that you take them on an empty stomach, take them 30 minutes to an hour before your first 10-Hour Coffee Diet coffee if possible, or between the coffees later in the day.

With this alternative, you will gain the advantages of that extended fasting while still controlling hunger due to the nutrients in the 10-Hour Coffee Diet coffee. But as amazing as this can be, your body is designed to eat real food. The extended modified fast ramps up a lot of good things and maximizes your body's potential for fat loss.

You are likely to enter a state known as "ketosis" where your fat burning kicks into high gear. You won't feel hungry using this protocol as long as you have 4 of the coffees. This version is easily the fastest way to drop a lot of fat. If you want fast and dramatic fat loss, use this version.

But again, use this infrequently due to the lack of variety in what and where you get your nutrients. I don't want you to risk having a nutrient deficiency by over-use of this timing protocol.

Alternative #9: If Muscle Building is Your Primary Goal (Extra Butter, Coconut Oil, and Protein Powder)

If your goal is to build muscle, and especially if you're performing weight-bearing exercises, this alternative protocol is the one for you.

To move the coffees more into helping you gain muscle (while still not gaining fat), add one extra tablespoon of butter, one extra tablespoon of coconut oil, and one extra serving (another 20 grams of protein) of protein powder to each coffee.

What works best is to have three of these coffees a day and one to two meals. Don't expect to get huge overnight the way so many claims are made when muscle gain is mentioned. You should definitely see improvement, however, and sometimes rapidly. The added calories from the healthy fats aid in your muscle gain, but that alone doesn't make it a quick process.

So, each coffee (up to 15 ounces) in this version would now have 2 to 2.5 tablespoons of grass-fed butter, 2 to 2.5 tablespoons of extra virgin organic coconut oil, and 40 grams of protein from protein powder. If you want to add another 4 to 8 ounces of almond milk into each coffee, you can still do that, too.

> **Note:** Given the extra healthy fats from the extra tablespoon of grass-fed butter and extra tablespoon of coconut oil, it's probably best to take a digestive supplement, like the NOW Super Enzymes that I discussed previously to help you digest the added fat when using this protocol.

You Can Overeat and Still Be Hungry

If you eat and drink fewer total calories than your body requires while getting all the necessary good fats and proteins (this is easy to do with high quality foods), you will lose fat at a fairly consistent pace.

The problem often is this: people get in the habit of eating a lot of low-quality foods such as chips and packaged sandwiches and boxed meals. Those essentially starve your body of nutrients it needs. More accurately, they don't *replace* the nutrients your body uses on a daily basis, leaving you in a nutrient-starved state. This makes your body crave more food which leads to overeating because the body is hungry for the missing nutrients. Starchy carbs are bad and lead almost to an instant hunger. Have you ever been able to eat "just a couple" good French fries or potato chips?

So your body ends up searching and craving more foods and more calories. The cycle grows.

If you begin upgrading the quality of your diet, especially with colorful vegetables (organic when you can) and grass-fed meat and good fats, you'll feed your body what it needs and you'll stop wanting to overeat. To help you achieve that, especially during the fasting part of your 10-Hour Coffee Diet, the grass-fed butter, organic extra virgin coconut oil or MCT oil, and the quality protein powder used in these specialized coffees, feed your body high quality fats and protein. They enable your body to function optimally and at a high level on fewer calories.

The results are better health and weight loss in the form of fat reduction. You should start craving far less food the better you eat.

Exercise Timing

Research suggests that at least 80% of weight loss directly relates to food you eat and not to exercise. You simply cannot burn enough calories to burn off fat and still eat badly. Conversely, those people who never exercise find that they can lose fat by changing the way they eat.

Obviously, exercise does help you lose weight and keep it off as well as provides a lot of positive strength and lifestyle benefits. Plus, we generally feel good once we get into a regular exercise routine.

Although this isn't primarily an exercise book, I suggest you do both weight-bearing exercises (such as using weights) as well as cardio exercises on an interval schedule. By that I mean they should be high intensity... such as intense running (not casual jogging) and then walking. Repeat that running-walking sequence 7 to 8 times.

There are two ideal times to exercise while on the 10-Hour Coffee Diet.

The best time is to exercise right before you eat your meal. The reason why is because the exercising (specifically if it's intense enough) will put your body into a hyper-state of nutrient hoarding. In this state the body sucks up all available calories to help repair the body. If you eat something within an hour after exercising, the easiest and most available calories your body will go after to use will be the ones flooding into your body after your meal.

Exercising before you eat is also a beneficial time because your body becomes extremely efficient at utilizing even the bad calories from the meal that you then eat. In other words, if you're going to eat something bad, make sure to do it within an hour after you've exercised.

The second best time to exercise is either immediately before drinking a 10-Hour Coffee Diet coffee or during one, meaning that you sip it throughout your routine. To me, this means a cold coffee of course because a hot version just isn't something you'll generally want during exercise.

Exercise traumatizes your muscles (that sounds dramatic, but it's a positive thing). To recover from the trauma the muscles could use some protein (muscles are made of protein). The protein speeds up your recovery from the "trauma" that the workout caused.

Silencing the Critics

I want to stop right here and make a quick point to which I have no doubt critics of this diet will say.

Some people might say this diet is a "fad" diet that would cause nutritional deficiencies if used over a year as outlined. To that I say the following: first, each individual can use the coffee diet as often or as little as they want. I offered many different variations to help fit the unique needs of each person. Unlike so many other diets, you are in control here. This is not a forced, one-size-fits-all program.

In addition, let's be honest. The two meals a day people skip in favor of the 10-Hour Coffee Diet coffees are most likely not healthy meals with *real* foods. They may look like real foods, but they're dead nutritionally. Those meals are mostly empty man-made calories that are making people more unhealthy and fatter.

I believe in you. I believe that you have common sense. Use the 10-Hour Coffee Diet plan as it suits your needs. If you are unsure about it, you are free to use it less often. As with any major change, it's always wise to consult a doctor first.

> **Note:** I never want to be disrespectful but most doctors seem to be completely illiterate when it comes to nutrition and natural health. Medicines and surgery are not always the answer. The tremendous death rate numbers from medicines given in hospitals, for example, the very buildings where medical knowledge should be supreme, are staggering.[45]

6

THE ACTUAL (LOW) COST OF THE 10-HOUR COFFEE DIET AND NUTRIENT MACRO INFORMATION

I suspect you'll be surprised at how much money you can save while losing weight and getting healthier on the 10-Hour Coffee Diet.

While this chapter might be one of the shorter chapters in the book, in many ways it's one of the most important to readers. You want to be able to afford a new eating plan such as the 10-Hour Coffee Diet and I'll present some numbers here to show you that it's extremely cost-effective. After I lay out the financial cost savings with the 10-Hour Coffee Diet, I'll also give you a rough estimated of the fat, protein, carbs, and calories you'll take in while on this diet.

Before beginning, you might already realize that intermittent fasting will save you tons on your groceries. Given that the best of the alternatives require just one full meal a day, the daily cost for the supplements and coffee is minimal. It's always nice to learn that getting healthier and leaner can also save you money, too.

Estimates of Course

The costs I present below are obviously estimates only. For each person reading, the costs will vary. In addition, the reading audience is international so your country may have far less costly supplements or coffee available while others may find that things cost more.

So the bottom line is this: If your prices for following the 10-Hour Coffee Diet are higher than these costs below, your savings on food that offset your higher costs will most likely also be higher because your food costs are most likely higher. In other words, your relative cost savings should mirror that of the cost savings below. It's my strong opinion that anybody anywhere can save a lot of money if they follow the 10-Hour Coffee Diet.

> **Note:** Any time somebody makes estimates they have to make assumptions. As I indicate above, use this chapter as a guideline to the relative costs you'll face. Since I try to use Amazon products everywhere I can, and since most people who are reading this most likely bought if from Amazon, you should easily be able to figure your own savings by locating the same or similar products on your nation's Amazon site if you're not in the USA.

The Base of the Estimates: Costing the Primary 10-Hour Coffee Diet Protocol

The following estimates come from the traditional 10-Hour Coffee Diet where you drink 2 coffees and have 1 meal. Since the meal will be the same cost for both your normal diet and the coffee diet, that is not factored in. For each of the two meals you're not eating, I will estimate each one costs $6. Again, this can vary widely from person to person. If your average cost per meal is more than $6 you will save even more money. If your costs are less, obviously you will save less money. But even then your savings on the 10-Hour Coffee Diet Plan will be proportionally the same.

Setting Up for Costing

If you follow the original 10-Hour Coffee Diet plan and follow the diet six days a week, that means about 26 days each month where you don't eat two of your regular full meals. So 26 days times 2 meals equals 52 meals you won't eat for most months on the plan. (And fortunately, you shouldn't be hungry either!)

Estimating that your average meal cost (meaning for breakfast and lunch) is about $6, the total you save equals about $312 each month ($312 = $6 times 52). That's huge! Sure, some days will cost you less and some more. And you can adjust down or up as you feel the need to do. Obviously the coffee and the 3 Weird Tricks are going to add back in some cost and we'll get there next.

But assuming the cost estimates above is about right for you, could you use an extra $312 each month?

Monthly Organic Coffee Costs

I listed coffees earlier that are cost-effective on Amazon. Here is a high quality, organic coffee. Amazon offers a 3-pack of it for just under $21 (obviously the price is subject to change, so I can't guarantee it remains that low).

This is pre-ground coffee, but let's face it, the easier it is to start something, the easier it will be to continue it. You don't need to grind beans, you don't need to drive to the store, just let Amazon bring it to your front door.

Here is the link to the Cafe Altura 3-pack: amazon.com/Cafe-Altura-Organic-Regular-12-Ounce/dp/B001EO772A/

Again, you don't need to buy this Cafe Altura brand if you don't want to. I've used it and I think it's one of the best values around (I'm a coffee snob and it tastes good to me too!). Using this coffee as an example, you get 36-ounces of organic coffee, or 1,017 grams of coffee.

If you're using two tablespoons per coffee (two tablespoons equal 28 grams) and two coffees each day, you will use about 56 grams of coffee a day. 1,017 grams divided by 56 daily grams equates to just over 18 days. So, that $21 worth of coffee will last you 18 days.

> **Note:** Bear with me on the math!

So, if you need enough coffee to last 26 days each month, you will need to get a second 3-pack for $21 and use up just under half of the second one. (You'll use the other half the next month). So, that adds another $10 to your monthly coffee costs.

Therefore, this pre-ground, good tasting, organic coffee each month is therefore about $31.

Monthly Organic Extra Virgin Coconut Oil Costs

Again, I'll assume you will use the standard two 10-Hour Coffee Diet coffees a day for about 26 days a month. At one tablespoon of coconut oil used for each of the monthly 52 coffees, you will need about 52 ounces of organic extra virgin coconut oil a month.

Here is the Amazon link for the organic extra virgin coconut oil that I suggested earlier in the book: amazon.com/Nutiva-Certified-Organic-Virgin-Coconut/dp/B000GAT6NG/

So, you will basically need the whole jar for the month. The total cost for your organic extra virgin coconut oil each month will be about $24.

> **Note:** If you instead will use the MCT Oil, the NOW brand is $21 for 32 ounces on Amazon here: amazon.com/NOW-Foods-100%25-32-Fluid-Ounces/dp/B0019LRY8A/
>
> You will need about 1.5 of those MCT Oil bottles per month. This makes your total monthly cost about $32. Remember, MCT Oil is better for mixing directly into the coffees, especially if you're adding in a cold liquid such as almond milk or pre-made cold coffee, but coconut oil is more versatile. I personally recommend the coconut oil due to both its lower cost and its better versatility in cooking.

If you have a Costco nearby, see if they have coconut oil. I recently bought their Carrington Farms Organic Extra Virgin Coconut oil, 54-ounces, for just $15.60... An $8 to $9 savings! Don't be afraid to look around and buy a brand not mentioned here.

Monthly Protein Powder Costs

I will use Optimum Nutrition's Gold Standard 100% Whey Protein at $53.99 for 5 pounds (as I write this) on Amazon. I mentioned it in an earlier chapter. You don't have to use this brand or even whey protein. Just note that you absolutely should *not* ever use soy protein powder because unfermented soy is an endocrine disruptor.

A link to the cookies & cream flavor is here: amazon.com/Optimum-Nutrition-Standard-Cookies-Cream/dp/B000GIPJZ2

You can choose whichever flavor you want. There are many different flavors to choose from and some of the numbers may vary slightly, but generally speaking, each flavor has 73-74 servings of 24 grams of protein. The flavors do not affect the nutrition or quality of the powders.

So, to get the total amount of grams we multiply 74 servings times 24 grams (the amount of protein in each serving). Please note that the total amount of grams per serving (about 30) also includes grams from carbs and fat. Don't pay attention to that number. Pay attention to only the protein grams. The 74 servings times 24 grams of protein per serving equals 1,776 grams of protein. I do not recommend you use the full serving of 24 grams of protein for each 10-Hour Coffee Diet coffee. I recommend about 20 grams of protein per coffee. So, this will be a little less than a scoop per serving for each coffee. (You will need to eyeball how much you put into each coffee. You won't be exact and that's okay. Don't worry about being exact.)

We take the 1,776 grams in the container and divide it by 20 (the amount of protein you'll use with each coffee). This equals just under 89 servings. So you have enough protein powder to last you for 89 coffees.

To find out the cost of the protein per month I'll need to divide the $54 cost of the protein powder by 89 coffees. The protein will cost 60-cents for each coffee. Multiply that by 52 coffees in a month (26 coffee days times 2 coffees a day) and the total cost for protein per month to you is about $31. You will also have enough left over protein powder to last you another 3 weeks.

These calculations don't factor in whether or not you drink the 10-Hour Coffee Diet coffees on your off days (once a week, or about 4-5 days each month).

Monthly Grass-Fed Butter Costs

Due to the shipping costs, it's not practical to buy butter from Amazon. The cost of Kerrygold Pure Irish Butter (unsalted) at Whole Foods is $2.99 for 8 ounces (it may cost more where you live). 8 ounces has 16 tablespoons of butter in it.

Because you are using one tablespoon of butter with each of the 52 coffees in the month you will need 52 tablespoons of butter, or 3 and a quarter bars of the Kerrygold grass-fed butter.

So, three bars of butter times $3 each is $9. Add another $1 for the quarter bar and we're up to $10 of butter needed for the month.

Note: ~~Good~~ news! We're almost done with all the math.

Concluding Numbers

Using my estimates above (most likely they will vary slightly from what you actually pay. Again, if you're not in the USA you'll obviously have to rework the numbers in your currency), here are the total costs to have these coffees each month.

Organic Coffee........................... $31

Organic Extra Virgin Coconut Oil... $24

Protein Powder.......................... $31

Grass-fed Butter........................ $10

Your total costs for the essential ingredients in these coffees is $96.

The 52 meals these coffees will be replacing would've cost you $312. $312 minus $96 equals $216 in monthly cost savings to you. $2,592 in savings over a year without starving yourself, with amazing fat loss, and with the health benefits that intermittent fasting provides!

And guess what? Not only are you working to improve your health factors, you upgraded the quality of what you're putting into your body. You save all that money while also adding three organic foods into your diet: Organic coffee, organic coconut oil, and organic butter.

I realize I keep coming back to relative costs, but this level of savings makes it too critical not to revisit. If you don't use the brands I used in the above calculations or if you're not in the USA, these items may cost you more. Still, saving a relative $100 each month on this diet is a deal anywhere on earth.

Stevia

If you choose to use Stevia sweetener, it won't change any protocol or the recipe for the 10-Hour Coffee Diet coffee. As stated earlier, you can add the Stevia whenever you want, even in the final cup before you take a sip.

Here is a link to the Kal Stevia that I suggested earlier: amazon.com/Kal-Pure-Stevia-Extract-Powder/dp/B000VRSR84

It costs $21.49 (as I write this) and will probably last you 3 to 4 months, more if you sprinkle just a little into each coffee. This makes the daily cost negligible (about 18-cents a day).

Note: The Stevia you end up using may or may not dissolve as easily as other kinds. If you find it difficult to stir your Stevia into the 10-Hour Coffee Diet coffee, sprinkle your Stevia into the coffee when it's in the blender, before blending. This allows the blender's action to do the stirring for you. This is the way I always do it.

If you want Stevia packets, consider getting NuStevia here: amazon.com/NuNaturals-Nustevia-Nocarbs-Blend-Packets/dp/B0019LWUJI

Unsweetened Almond Milk

In your local grocery store, you can find conventional almond milk (often called *Almond Breeze* or *Almond Drink* or *Silky Almond*) for about $2.78 for a half gallon. If you use 5 ounces in each coffee, this will last you about a week.

I don't like hot drinks. I use the almond milk to cool off the coffee. It also gives it a nice texture, at least for me. It has very few calories (30 calories per 8 ounces) and is healthy. Feel free to use 4-8 ounces of almond milk with your 10-Hour Coffee Diet coffee.

Macro Information – The Coffee's "Cost" in Calories

A book such as this one wouldn't be complete without giving you the primary caloric and nutritional counts (also called "macros") of the ingredients used most.

Protein Powder

Each serving of protein powder has the 24 grams of protein, 1.5 grams of fat, 3 grams of carbohydrates, and is 120 calories. You typically won't use the whole serving. You're aiming for approximately 20 grams of protein.

In general, this means you'll end up getting about 100 calories, 20 grams of protein, a little over 1 gram of fat, and about 2.5 grams of carbohydrates.

Organic Extra Virgin Coconut Oil

Each tablespoon serving you take with your coffee has 130 calories and 14 grams of healthy fats.

Grass-Fed Butter

Each tablespoon of butter you take with the coffee has 100 calories and 12 grams of healthy fat.

The Combined Macros for Each Coffee

You will end up getting about 330 calories, 20 grams of protein, 27 grams of fat (it's healthy fat remember), and about 2.5 grams of carbohydrates from each coffee.

7

10-HOUR COFFEE DIET Q&A'S

I'll close out this 10-Hour Coffee Diet section of the book with a few common answers to questions that arise from time to time.

Q: I prefer tea to coffee. Can I replace the coffee with tea and still get the benefits of the 10-Hour Coffee Diet plan?

A: Yes. We've had testers extensively test using tea instead of coffee. It works, however the taste is much more bland than using coffee. I prefer you stick with coffee, but you do have the option to switch it out and use tea instead.

I suggest you try yerba mate tea due to its somewhat extra metabolic push, such as this organic yerba mate box of 25 tea bags from Amazon ($7) here:

amazon.com/Guayaki-Yerba-Mate-Organic-25-Count/dp/B008234L0C/

Of course just use your own favorite tea if you have one. I always prefer organic over conventional, but conventional tea will give you most of the same fat loss benefits as organic. Green tea also provides extra health benefits over black tea[46] but again, let taste and cost guide you.

You can follow every one of the alternative protocols using the tea instead of coffee. For some, a creamy tea doesn't taste as good as a creamy coffee, so try the 10-Hour Coffee Diet's coffee recipe using tea and see what you think. There's no inherent problem with swapping the coffee for the tea. If you don't like the taste, then go back to using coffee.

Q: I find this far easier than I expected! What happens if I decide to follow the 10-Hour Coffee Diet every day of the week?

A: There's nothing unhealthy about the plan and you can follow it every day. The benefits of the intermittent fasting with the modified 24-hour fast elements combine to do your body a lot of good.

A big key is whether or not the food you eat is, for the most part, healthy. You need to make sure you're giving your body all the fuel it needs through a variety of foods so you're consuming a variety of nutrients. Processed foods (fake foods) contain little or no nutrients. I don't want you to just lose weight. I want you to also be as healthy as possible.

Over a period of weeks, your body changes the way it works with a hormone known as *leptin*[47] if you eat fewer meals too often. In general, once a week you should eat more than one meal while on this plan. Doing so helps keep your leptin in check. Your body actually gets fooled into not knowing if food will be coming in single meals or multiple meals if you eat multiple meals one day a week. Your body will self-regulate its leptin better this way.

Basically, once a week you can cheat if you feel the need. Just don't cheat and have a bunch of pasta and dessert if you don't really want it. Also, don't pig out. If you don't want to cheat and if you want to stay on the plan, on the seventh day just make sure to use a version of the plan that entails 2 meals for the day. Consider the seventh day each week as a free day. I recommend that you increase your calories and eat at least 2 meals that day.

Q: I keep forgetting to get the timing right. How can I keep track of when to drink each coffee?

A: Don't worry about it too much. You don't need to be precise. The worst case scenario is your body will let you know when it needs another coffee.

Q: What if I get hungry?

A: If you get hungry any time before your meal, immediately drink at least 8 ounces of filtered water or plain tea. This is often enough to tide you over until the next coffee or meal.

Q: How much weight could I expect to lose?

A: You won't like the answer, but honestly, it's different for each person. Each person is different so each person will get different results. I don't know how dedicated you'll be using the diet. I don't know how much weight you need to lose (people who have more weight to lose obviously lose more weight initially).

I don't know if you've had surgery or use medicines or if you have hormonal problems or an imbalance in brain neurotransmitters, and so on.

Q: Can I use more or less water for the coffees than what you recommend?

A: Yes. Start with the recommended amount for the first few days and feel free to adjust from there.

Q: I tried the 10-Hour Coffee Diet coffee and didn't like the taste. How can I improve it?

A: You can basically do 4 things. First, you can use stevia to sweeten it up. I personally use 2 stevia packets. Second, you can use more coffee. I use 2 tablespoons for each 15 ounces of coffee. However much coffee you personally use, add 1 more tablespoon and see how that goes. Third, you can increase the amount of protein powder you use by 10 grams. Fourth, sprinkle in some cinnamon.

Q: Will this work if I don't use organic coffee... or grass-fed butter... or organic extra virgin coconut oil?

A: A better question is if it will work as well. The answer is, no, it won't work as well. Not even close. Don't be cheap. Use the high quality products recommended (or something of similar quality). You'll still end up saving a lot of money from your monthly food expenses. We had dozens of testers and all of them tested using regular coffee, regular butter, and non-organic coconut oil. There's a reason why we recommend the products that we do. You're free to use regular products. Just don't complain and say *The 10-Hour Coffee Diet* doesn't work if you're not happy with the results.

Q: I want to lose fat as fast as possible. How often can I use the variation of *The 10-Hour Coffee Diet* where I don't eat any food for 1-3 days and only drink 3-4 coffees per day?

A: I'm always concerned when a person doesn't get nutrients from a variety of sources due to a lack of variety in their diet because over time they'll develop some sort of nutrient deficiency. Because of that I recommend that you use the no-food variation of the diet no more than 3 days each week so that the risk of any sort of nutrient deficiency is minimized. You can do it 3 days in a row or every other day for up to 3 days in a week. So, up to 3 days a week is the answer. You can do that for weeks or months at a time.

Also note that you can do the other variations of *The 10-Hour Coffee Diet* that require you to eat food the rest of the week. Just remember to pay attention to your body and use commonsense if you feel sick from a lack of food. It's usually just the body's way of adjusting. Now, could you use the no-food version of the diet more than 3 days a week? Yes, you can. But I don't feel comfortable recommending that without knowing you and your personal health history. In fact, if you do in fact do this version of the diet 3 days in a week, I'd much rather you wait a full week before doing it again.

Q: This isn't really a fast, is it?

A: No. This is a modified fast; although I'm sure technical people would argue the point. A true fast doesn't allow you to have fats or proteins... or any calories for the matter. While a true water-only fast does have health benefits, a modified fast that allows for healthy fats and proteins (and food) is better able to maintain brain health (the brain is made of fats), your metabolism (starving causes your body to go into a catabolic state and eat your muscles for energy and thus causes your metabolism to slow down because muscle burns off more calories than body fat), and your sanity (*The 10-Hour Coffee Diet* is pleasant and easy to do, a water fast not so much).

Q: Is this similar to David Asprey's BP coffee?

A: David Asprey's ideas on coffee were an inspiration and *The 10-Hour Coffee Diet* coffees are similar in nature to his BP coffee. However, for optimal health and weight loss *The 10-Hour Coffee Diet* coffees and the flexibility of our various timing protocols can't be beat for overall health and weight loss.

Q: Does the heat from the coffee degrade the benefits of the protein from the protein powder?

A: Heat does affect it. Although some peptides denature between 158-176 degrees Fahrenheit, the amino acid profile stays the same. Bottom line? You have nothing to worry about. The heat from the coffee won't compromise the protein powder.

Q: Can kids drink *The 10-Hour Coffee Diet* coffees? Are they safe and healthy for them?

A: Is organic coffee healthier than sodas and Kool-Aid? Is grass-fed butter healthy? Is Extra Virgin organic coconut oil healthy? Is a little bit extra protein through protein powder good for growing kids? The answer to all those questions is YES.

You'd be doing a world of good for your kids if you switched out sodas and Kool-Aid for 1-2 of *The 10-Hour Coffee Diet* coffees each day. Since children are still growing I would advise against using the timing protocols and instead have them eat like normal. If they drink soda or Kool-Aid with their meals, instead use a *10-Hour Coffee Diet* coffee and see if they like it. You may also want to use less butter, less coconut oil, less protein powder, and less coffee.

If you are worried or uncomfortable about giving your kids a *10-Hour Coffee Diet* coffee, then don't. I understand there are people who have no problem giving their kids McDonald's and sodas but freak out at the thought of children drinking coffee, or in this case coffee with healthy fats and protein added to it. We can't please everyone. So we won't even try. If they want to criticize, let them. We would never recommend something that is unhealthy and unsafe for children (or you)!

Q: I'm no longer happy with the rate at which I'm losing weight... what can I do?

A: First, try switching to a different timing protocol. Perhaps use the protocol where you fast using just the *10-Hour Coffee Diet* coffees for 1-3 days without eating any food. If you're using coconut oil, switch to using MCT oil. If you're using MCT oil, switch to using coconut oil.

Section 2

–

Brain Controlled Weight Loss – The Solution to Failed Diets & Exercise Programs!

8

INTRODUCING THE BRAIN CONTROLLED WEIGHT LOSS PROGRAM

Now that you know the specifics about the 10-Hour Coffee Diet I want to dig deeper into a more holistic approach to health and weight loss. I want you to take an approach to your health that goes beyond simply following a diet or exercising.

Don't we constantly lament how wonderful it would be if only we could get our body in shape and working well again? Then maybe we'd feel well enough to fix some of the other baggage we have such as our emotional roadblocks, our restless sleep, our fading personal relationships... you know all those non-physical things that bug us almost as much as our bodies bug us.

The problem is that we often put the cart before the horse.

I am about to expose some insights into the mind-body connection that many of you have never known before. People are stunned to learn that a lot of our health and body problems are rooted in our brain.

If you continuously struggle with your health and weight loss, you'd be wise to focus on your brain first!

Fix the Brain, Fix the Body, Fix the Baggage

The brain is the ultimate control center. Your brain, your body's central processing unit, controls often overrides all other factors on how fast you lose or gain weight, how good or bad you feel, and how your body turns the food you give it into fat or fuel.

Ultimately the health of your brain determines the health of your body.

With the first section of this book, you learned how to feed your body is an extremely optimal way. The 10-Hour Coffee Diet's coffees and eating schedule is one of the most powerful combinations ever devised for ramping up your fat loss and lean muscle retention. But even on that plan, your body might not lose as much fat as it could... and if that's the case, the answer is almost always found in your brain… not your stomach!

Coffee and Your Brain

Here's the great news about getting your brain in gear. The requirements for improving your brain go hand-in-hand with every technique found in the 10-Hour Coffee Diet. All of the supplements that go into your coffee drinks as well as the food I suggested for your meals align with fantastic brain health. The 10-Hour Coffee Diet speeds your brain's recovery as you move forward.

You must here and now make a promise to yourself: Assuming I convince you that the proper brain fuel produces the best body results possible, and I will, your goal from this point forward should be to focus on your brain and also your stomach.

You've been sold a bill of goods all your life when you've been told that to lose weight and build lean muscle mass, get more energy, and feel better, that you have to fix your body. Not so. To the extent you've happened to fix your brain in the past you may have accomplished all those things, but since you didn't realize the prime importance of focusing on your brain first you didn't accomplish your goals as fully as you could have. And if you're like most of us, you didn't stay lean or feel good for long. Because you weren't taught that your brain is the organ you should make as healthy as possible and then your brain will take care of the rest of you.

Fix your brain; fix your body. This is the solution to failed diets and failed exercise programs.

Let's get to it.

9

THE BRAIN AND BODY TRINITY: FOOD, SUPPLEMENTS, AND DRUGS

To make your brain work for you, and therefore to have the healthiest body you can achieve, you must give your brain the nutrients it requires. Doing so stimulates brain chemicals that go to work putting you back in balance, both emotionally as well as physically.

There are three ways to give your brain what it needs:

1. Food
2. Supplements
3. Drugs

I'm not as thrilled about #3 as I am the others, but I also realize medicine has a vital place in our health. Primarily, medicine used to repair problems is a must. It's the long-term preventative meds that I am wary of. Long-term medicines such as statins to control cholesterol (cholesterol has gotten a bad rap) seem to be less effective and more dangerous than at least *trying* one of the numerous ways of controlling cholesterol through diet, supplementation, and of course exercise. I encourage you to focus less on prescription drugs to put your brain or body into the balance it needs and more on supplements and diet. At least give it a try before going the prescription route.

Note: I truly am not anti-drug. It's true that sometimes we break a bone or we are severely injured or we happen to get so sick so quickly, through infection from another person, that a natural food or supplement remedy simply won't have enough time to work before it's too late for us. I am, however, anti-drug for general health and fitness and for minor illnesses that everybody experiences and gets over if they treat the illness properly.

We're mostly going to focus on food and supplements in this section. It might surprise you that our preference is that we get *all* our nutrients from our food. But that is not always possible. So we will look both to food and supplements to maximize our brains and then from there our bodies become healthier and the weight loss process unlocked.

Food Isn't What It Used to Be

Our food supply has lost many of its nutrients through over-farming the same land, using genetically-altered seeds that produce less-than the highest quality food, the overuse of pesticides, the over-application of fertilizers, and so on.

One reason organic food these days sells fairly well, in spite of the fact it lasts half as long as non-organic and costs twice as much is that organic food is grown without the growth hormones and the pesticides that invaded virtually everything in the grocery's produce section. In addition, organic food should have more nutrients given that its soil must be richer with minerals in order for it to survive without the chemical treatments used on other foods. The more nutrients produced, the less bugs will want it.

Eating organic foods automatically makes you eat less because organic foods provide you with more nutrients. Your body doesn't feel starved for nutrients. You are less likely to chase after more and more food from incorrect cravings for bad foods and the low-nutrients found in non-organic products (called *conventional* foods).

Our meat supplies haven't fared much better than non-organic conventional produce either. The chickens we eat are raised in giant buildings where they stay within the same square foot or so of space their entire lives, pooping where they stand and sleep, and being fed corn laced with antibiotics to keep them from getting deathly ill and dying after birth from that environment. Our meat supply is similar with our cattle being fed antibiotic-laced corn grain their entire lives. The grain is also laced with growth hormones to falsely grow the animals faster and fatter to get them to slaughter as quickly as possible.

Eating grain is unnatural for cattle. Cattle were made to eat grass.

I'm not giving away any industry secrets here, although the produce, beef, and chicken industries sure wish all this information were secret. The knowledge of the way most of our food is grown is why in specialized supermarkets and online you can find healthy grass-fed beef from cattle raised without hormones and that grazed in fields most of their lives. You can find cage-free chickens and eggs from hens that roamed the grounds of the farms, eating bugs and other gooey things that are good for them. You can find pork that was raised in a free-range situation and Wild Alaskan Salmon that was not farm-raised for the same reasons and that also have virtually no toxic mercury that stays in your body harming your cells.

Please understand this isn't an all-or-nothing proposition. You don't have to eat only organic foods. And you certainly don't have to put a chicken coop on your driveway for eggs! Everything you do to make improvements, a little at a time, builds upon the last thing you did. Eventually you may find that you feel so much better as you make small changes that you decide to continue making more. This positive feedback happens to all of us; it's surprising how small changes can make a big difference in the way we feel and the way our brains function.

Dr. Al Sears, MD, wrote this:

> *You've heard the saying about "an apple a day," right? My granddad told me that when I was a kid. He lived into his 90s and was as strong as an ox up until the day he died. But today an apple a day is not going to do anything for you.*
>
> *The produce you get from your grocery store doesn't have the same level of vitamins, minerals or fiber it did years ago. In fact, you would have to eat* ***26 of today's apples to equal just one apple from 1914.***[48]

Why should you care about that? A lot of commercial farming has stripped our food of the very nutrients we need to stay vital, young and full of energy.

Today's commercial farmers grow fruits and vegetables that are designed to look good on the shelf. That means they're often little more than pith and water. And harsh fertilizers leave the soil with few – if any – minerals to nourish the plants.

Even the U.S. Department of Agriculture admits that vitamin and mineral levels have fallen by as much as 81 percent over the last 30 years.[49]

Are You Willing to Pay the Price?

All the good and healthy food sources cost more because it costs money to raise food the right way. But that's the price we pay to be healthy. I'm assuming you know better than to raise children on three meals a day of Krispy Kreme donuts. (I love Krispy Kreme by the way! But it's a *very* rare treat, if in fact it should be called a treat.) But if you did feed your children only Krispy Kreme donuts, it would sure be less expensive than giving them meat and vegetables. So, you already know that you must pay what it takes to get nutrition. And I suggest that you begin looking at your food sources, and checking local farms and farmer's markets, to see if you can supply your pantries and freezers with these kinds of items:

- Grass-fed, hormone-free, antibiotic-free beef (*)
- Free-range, cage-free chickens and eggs
- Free-range, hormone-free pork
- Free-range, hormone-free lamb
- Mercury-free wild Alaskan salmon
- Fresh, raw, whole milk (**)

* Eating grass-fed, hormone-free beef is far more important to me than buying from a strict "certified organic" beef. When a cow gets sick, and they do once in a while even in the cleanest and most careful of farms, they might need an injection of an antibiotic to get them well again... and that's okay. If the ranch or farm is certified "organic" they are not allowed to administer the antibiotic and the cow might die, thus raising your price since the herd will not be as full as it might otherwise be. You should always prefer certified organic fruit and vegetables compared to conventional produce, however, because antibiotics are not an issue there.

** If raw milk is legal in your state, you should consider using it exclusively. It not only tastes far better than store-bought milk, the homogenization and pasteurization from store-bought milk destroys all the natural and healthy nutrients from milk and changes the milk's structure which produces most cases of lactose intolerance found today. Stay away from skim milk of any kind, even raw skim milk, if you want to lose weight. Fat does not make you fat. Only bad fat makes you fat... such as the trans fats in hydrogenated vegetable oils.

You can often find healthy grass-fed, free-range meat sources through local farms, farmer's markets, and co-ops in your area. Check around and do some Internet searches. You'll find them. As long as you begin to veer away from packaged food, you're moving in the right direction even if you don't go all-in for grass-fed and organic produce.

You Can't Get Your Brain Fixed As Efficiently Through Food Alone

In spite of the wealth of information I just gave you about your food source, it is simply too difficult to get the nutrients you need from food alone these days. If possible, eat organic fruit and vegetables and get your meat and eggs sourced from farms and ranches that supply and raise animals the way I suggest above. But even then our ground has been reduced of its nutrients through runoff and through the lack of crop rotation on a wide-scale basis.

Some farmers are learning about a concept called *high brix* gardens. These are gardens grown with the maximum amount of nutrients possible through fixing the soil first before worrying about the plants. One of the pillars of the high brix community is International Ag labs[50] and you can learn all about this thing called a high brix garden there.

If you're willing to try, it is *easy* to grow a high-brix garden. You don't need much room to grow such a garden that will produce a lot of unbelievably tasty fruits and vegetables. Did you know that radishes and turnips, when grown properly, are sweet? Amazingly sweet. And that sweetness is the major indicator of their high brix nutrient content.

Supplements Are the Key Today

But let's face it. You're not going to grow your own produce by tomorrow. And you might not ever want to for a variety of reasons. If not, you are left with buying your food. Just make sure it's food that is as healthy as possible. Follow my recommendations above.

But even that food won't do it for your brain or body as quickly and as effectively as you'd like. You want to be healthy, lean, joyful, and on top of your game by tonight at midnight, right?

While that may be a little too much to expect, you *can* speed up the process by which you make your brain the healthiest it can be. While you should begin immediately changing your food supply, and we'll talk more about specific foods that fix your brain and body, the *best* way to tackle things fast is through supplements.

Supplements allow you to balance your body and brain quickly and efficiently. Much of the focus will be on the supplement aspect of the brain/body connection. We'll also discuss food quite a bit. By supplementing good food with even higher-nutrient-dense supplements, you stack your advantages far more. And you speed up the process by which your brain and body get into balance and into shape making you the best *you* possible.

The Brain Determines Your Weight Gain and Weight Loss

Mystery stories often wait until the final chapter, sometimes the final page, and even the final sentence to tell who did it.

Not here!

I'm going to tell you the answer before I show you the reasons why and the solutions on how to achieve it.

The answer is this: if you get your brain in balance, your body will follow. That means your health will begin to improve and not just your emotional and psychological health, but your physical health as well. In addition, you will lose weight. And I dare say, for those in the minority who need to gain weight, you will gain weight! Your mind has an uncanny ability to know what your normal state should be and will go to work immediately to achieve that normal state if you supply the right energy for it to do so.

As odd as it sounds, you lose weight *first* in your brain. Your brain then works on your body to bring it into alignment with weight loss. If you turn off the weight loss in your brain (or weight gain for those who genuinely need to gain weight), then it will work against your body. All of this occurs not just on a chemical level, although that is primary. All of this also occurs in other ways. Your brain, through the function of brain-related enzymes and chemicals, will turn on your satiation switch (telling yourself, "I'm full!") when it's properly functioning and will not turn it on or will delay it (telling yourself, "I need another half-gallon of mint chocolate chip ice cream!") when your brain is out of whack.

Where your brain goes, your body follows.

Turning On the Juice

The chemicals in your mind are the catalyst but not the complete way your brain controls your body. Your brain is a lot like a computer's processing chip. That may be news to you. Your brain, like a computer, communicates with your body and does its job through the use of millions of tiny electrical pulses going to and from cells, across what is called synapses.

When your brain is out of balance, through bad nutrition for example, your brain's electrical charges don't function well. They are inefficient. Your mind's little switches switch more slowly than they otherwise would. You feel sluggish. You just want comfort foods, which in that situation, will almost always result in a high-carb, low-nutrition food such as fast food, dessert, French fries, or mashed potatoes and gravy with corn and deep-fried chicken. This is all food that brings about a false feeling of comfort.

> **Note:** The carbs in starchy foods like corn and potatoes, and sweets such as ice cream and fruit juices, do supply energy, but they do so via what is known as a "sugar high." Such energy is fleeting and quickly runs out leaving your brain far more sluggish than before you ate them. Protein-rich meals such as fish and grass-fed beef will give you far longer energy without an instant energy letdown. We'll talk more about how different kinds of foods affect you in a little bit.

And as you eat those foods, you feel like moving less. And your mind and body slow down more. And your brain's electrical impulses slow down further. And you feel more sluggish than before. And the carbs quickly turn to sugar and the sugar high quickly dies. And you begin craving more of the same food... and less activity and exercise and sun and fresh air. And your brain gets more sluggish. And the beat goes on.

But you can reverse that! *Today* you can begin to reverse that!

And I'm so sure of this that I'm telling you that if you begin to follow the suggestions outlined here your mind should begin to go back into a normal balance almost immediately. While it's true that some people can get so sick that they can't revert back to a healthy state quickly or ever, our bodies are amazing regeneration factories. Our cells actually replace themselves over and over throughout our lifetimes. And like the Six Million Dollar Man, "you can rebuild them" and you can begin rebuilding your cells right away.

You can turn the "juice" back on, you can flip your brain's switches from sluggish to efficient, and your brain will begin turning your body back into what it was designed to be: a lean, efficient, active, workhorse that you can utilize to do amazing things that right now you might feel are out of reach.

The Diet Mentality

In spite of this book's most critical first section about the 10-Hour Coffee Diet, I am going to get on your case a little about being on a "diet."

Yet in spite of them being called "diets," including my own 10-Hour Coffee diet, I will warn you against the traditional "going on a diet."

Such diets fail.

You know it and I know it. We both should admit what has happened every time you've gone on a diet. You've lost weight and then gained it all back and often more.

Crash diets and two hours of aerobics are sure recipes for waistline disaster.

Eating to feed your brain and therefore your body, as well as exercising in a smart way so you don't spend hours and hours in a gym each week, are the only ways to enjoy your life and like the way your body looks and feels.

> **Note:** As a matter of fact, the exact opposite of a "crash diet" might be required to begin balancing your brain and get your body into a fat-burning mode. You may very well have to begin eating more calories than you do now to get needed nutrients into your system so they begin to work. A calorie doesn't always seem to be a full calorie in the traditional sense. Your total daily calories may very well *increase* on the 10-Hour Coffee Diet. To lose weight it is the *type* of calorie you eat that determines whether a calorie easily adds to your fat cells or turns directly into energy that doesn't get stored. Most of the foods that your brain functions well on happen to be the very foods you can eat a lot of and yet they don't pack the pounds like the foods that are bad for your brain, even if you eat those brain foods in bigger quantities.

When your brain begins to become active, healthy, and efficient again, you will not ever again need to think about the word "diet" again. Your body will naturally begin craving more good foods. Your body will begin to appreciate and not dread activity once again.

A Healthy Brain Equals a Young Person

Fuel is needed for thinking, for feeling good, for rebuilding cells, for sleeping well, and for creating a "feel good" feeling that just won't go away.

Have you ever met two people about the same age but one looks and acts far more youthful while the other appears old? Do you know what the main difference between them usually is? The youthful person has a brain that is properly fueled. The older-seeming person has let her brain get out of sync and has nutritionally gone unbalanced.

A sluggish brain is an old brain.

Do you feel old before your time?

If you can fix your brain, your body will reverse in age faster than you ever thought possible.

> **Note:** A non-profit educational organization composed of nutritionists, doctors, psychiatrists, psychologists, and scientists called "Food for the Brain" recently published this statement leaving no doubt as to the link between nutrition and what was once thought to be genetic or just "old-timers" diseases (the boldfaced text is mine for emphasis): *The good news is that a number of encouraging research avenues indicate that dementia and Alzheimer's could be prevented, and possibly halted in the early stages by* ***a comprehensive optimum nutrition approach.*** *One of the reasons this is likely is that* ***only one in a hundred cases of Alzheimer's is caused by genes.*** *We also know that new brain cells are being made all the time, even in old age and, under the right conditions, new brain cell growth can be encouraged. Current research is focusing on how to encourage, not only, neuron growth, but also how to enhance the formation of new dendrite connections.* ***But the most exciting frontier is improving your nutrition to prevent memory decline in the first place.***

So literally, the more nutrition you give your brain the younger you will be. And when we think of someone who seems "older than their years," the odds are great that most or all of the symptoms that make them seem old are nutritional related.

Thorin Klosowski recently wrote: *According to Shukitt-Hale, certain foods can change gene expression in the brain and increase neuronal brain communication by creating new brain cells. It's thought that one food type that may help brain cell production comes from the fatty acid omega-3, which is found abundantly in fish and walnuts. Eating a serving of these every day in combination with exercise can help rebuild those brain cells.*[51]

It is no exaggeration to state that making our brains healthier through diet, supplements, and exercise *literally* makes us younger because our brains grow more cells, we feel younger, we live longer, and our cognitive skills are boosted.

Where Does Weight Loss Come Into the Picture?

I assume that most of you reading this book are doing so because you want to lose weight. Yeah, you also want to feel better and be healthier, but that is often our secondary goals in spite of them being so important. We want to look good!

I've already covered the failures of traditional diets, especially the horrid "crash diet." I want you convinced that a healthy lifestyle and not gimmick crash diets (yes we have written books on diets, but they aren't gimmicks… they are part of a healthy long term weight loss and maintenance strategy) is what we all need to maximize our brains and bodies. And if you have been told that you have a genetic predisposition to be overweight, I want you to know that nutrition trumps genes almost 100% of the time. Fix your nutrition and you fix your brain and you can forget all about the genetic baggage you may have been told about.

The genetic tendencies we all have, in one way or another, are simply indicators and slight nudges from lifestyle failures. Here is what I mean by that. If you come from a family of overweight people, then you have a tendency to choose and eat the kinds of foods that will continue that overweight condition in your life. That is why you are overweight in the vast majority of cases.

There is a strong environmental association that often belies the fact that many families do *not* have a genetic disposition towards obesity even if most of the members are obese. The environmental impact of growing up in families that had low activity levels, ate unhealthy foods, and knew or cared little about nutrition is going to be passed onto you. Learning what works and what does not, and learning how to fix your own brain, is one of the most beneficial ways you'll ever find to lose weight… even if you come from a family of obese relatives.

In spite of Grandma's wonderful waffles that gave her, her daughter, and her grandchildren big thighs and waists, you can instantly break that chain. You will find that almost certainly your genetics play a lesser role than you've been told all your life.

Cravings don't begin in your stomach or mouth. Your brain is where cravings begin.

Why Most Diets Fail – An Out-of-Balanced Brain Doesn't Have its Required Nutrients

May I tell you a story? It's a true story.

I have a friend named Bob whose sister was put in a hospital a few years back for what they called "mental dysfunction" of some kind. Bob and his mother went to the doctor to find out why he admitted his sister. She certainly had been acting strange for a while and not getting along well with the rest of the family so something was wrong. But the hospital admission seemed severe.

When the mom asked what the girl's problem was, the doctor replied, "She has a chemical imbalance."

The mother asked a very good question: "What chemical?"

The doctor's reaction to the question was: stunned silent ignorance.

After a long pause, the doctor began stammering and after a few grunts and "Ums," he finally asked, "What do you mean 'What chemical'?"

The mother said, "You said she had a chemical imbalance. I want to know what chemical is out of balance."

There was an even longer pause before the doctor said, "Well, there's not actually a specific chemical really, it's more of a... it's more of a behavioral issue and we can treat her with some drugs to help get her back into balance."

The mother said, "If it's not a chemical imbalance, why did you say she had a chemical imbalance?"

The doctor was noticeably upset with that line of questioning and began showing some anger. His voice's volume increased as he said, "It could be any number of things and we would like to keep her under observation until we know what is wrong."

Bob immediately marched into his sister's room and said this: "You are acting in a way that has been embarrassing to the family and everybody around you. I am ashamed of you. You need to act like a grown woman, begin taking care of yourself, and start respecting other people as much as you respect yourself. You often go around saying things like, 'people are so dumb' and 'I get tired of being around idiots all the time' and what you forget is that *you* are people too! You are in the human race and you accuse others of being jerks a lot while you are a jerk to almost everybody you interact with."

He stormed out of the room.

Let's face it... that sure sounds like a harsh thing to say to one's sister.

She jumped out of bed, ran out of the room, and hugged him, crying, and saying she was sorry and that he was correct! His words jolted her into reality. She didn't have a chemical problem in her brain. She had a thinking problem that needed to be dealt with and not coddled. The doctor would have preferred to medicate her for a week or two and drug her into submission. The family checked her out of the hospital right then and I saw a remarkable change take over her. She actually needed exactly what her brother said. It took the mother's brilliant and innocent question to trigger the brother's understanding of the whole thing.

Now why do I tell you that story? I am well aware of the fact that some people have severe mental problems that must be dealt with in a scientific and often a medical and also a nutritional way. And I realize that some might only get slightly better or never better depending on how far along they are and how severe the problem is. But that doesn't change the reality that many are put through the system that simply need to get their mind and their bodies back on track.

If a month at Psychology Drug & Resorts sounds good to you right now, you should consider the fact that you can probably do far more to fix your own brain than the "doctors" can do who throw meds at the problem, not knowing which "chemical" is the one that is out of balance.

It is Not Actually a Chemical Imbalance, but a Nutrition Imbalance

The ironic thing about the previous section is that many people do have a nutritional imbalance that affects their brain. We are going to discuss some very specific nutrients – here I go – actual *chemicals* that may be out of balance in your brain. But unlike the brain imbalance that they toss drugs at, these nutritional chemicals are easily balanced in most people through nutrition.

And the fastest and most effective ways to get those nutritional chemicals in balance is through food and supplementation. Not through random psycho drugs.

Your Brain Needs to Lose Weight

When you're overweight, your body isn't just fat on the outside. Your inside is fat too. Fat builds up all around your organs. This visceral fat encloses your heart, lungs, liver, and other internal organs. The fat keeps your cells from communicating effectively. The fat keeps your organs from functioning at their peak efficiency. This organ-enveloping fat keeps your body feeling old. And an old-feeling body *ages more rapidly than it would otherwise age.*

Your internal belly fat (called *omentum*) looks far worse than the fat that sticks out of your bikini!

Remember in the last chapter when we discussed how the brain communicates with itself and other organs in your body? It does so through electrical impulses. When your brain gets fat on the inside, as it and every other part of your body does when you're overweight, those electrical impulses are squeezed for space. They communicate far less efficiently. And normal healthy impulses from your brain such as the "I'm full" signal takes far longer to reach your craving center that makes you reach for the next Snickers bar... or keeps you *from* reaching for the next Snickers bar.

The Fantastic Four

Much of this book is going to focus on four brain nutrients that you must get in balance right away.

I call them the Fantastic Four because they are so amazing in how they change us for the good when balanced... or for the worse if they're out of balance.

The Fantastic Four brain chemicals are:

- Dopamine
- Serotonin
- GABA
- Acetylcholine

My friend's sister that was diagnosed with a "chemical imbalance" by that doctor who could not name *one brain chemical* that might have been out of balance... I suspect – and no, I am not a doctor and I don't play one in books – I suspect that my friend had an imbalance of dopamine, serotonin, GABA, and acetylcholine. She probably was not out of balance of all four, but at least one.

Plus, she was emotionally out of balance because everybody walked on eggshells around her instead of helping her by telling her the direct truth. I knew her well and what her brother told her was something all of us wanted to say at one time or another: "I am ashamed of the way you're behaving."

And his words were honest. He used no malice. He spoke the truth. And she responded. After that she was a completely changed individual. She also asked me to help her lose weight. I told her I'd be thrilled to help her. And we began working on her lifestyle even though she asked for a diet.

Although I've since learned to fix the brain before the muscles, the foods that I told her to eat happened to be the very foods that put into balance everyone's brain chemical nutrients: dopamine, serotonin, GABA, and acetylcholine.

Good nutrition fixes problems.

Bad Nutrition – Problems Are Waiting in the Wings

Your number one enemy is sugar.

This means sugar. This means High Fructose Corn Syrup. This means honey. Yes, this even means fruit in most forms.

While real honey and fruit aren't dangerous or your enemy in and of themselves, they are almost always used in such a way that they become just as much of your enemy as processed, white sugar. And if processed, white sugar is bad, High Fructose Corn Syrup is worse. And it is virtually impossible for you to eat any food bought today that doesn't contain sugar in one form or another.

> **Note:** If an ingredient ends in *–ose*, just assume it is sugar. It might be called sucrose or dextrose or glucose or fructose, but it's sugar. A cream-filled donut by any other name tastes just as sweet and harms your brain just as much.

What About Fat, Eggs, Milk, and Red Meats?

The damage that sugar and sugar substitutes do to your brain first, and then your body, is so great that even the government's FDA will admit eating too much sugar is bad for you. Their food pyramid has been a complex system of pretty bad advice.

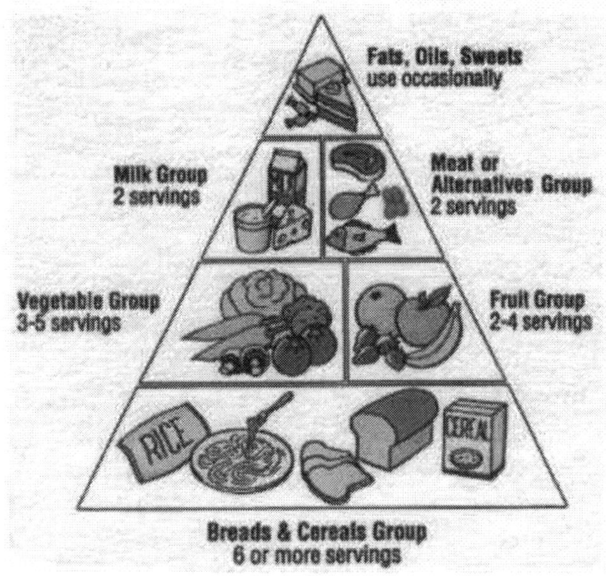

The food ideas promoted literally say: eat more unhealthy foods than healthy foods.

If this surprises you, please understand that grains, the entire bottom layer of the FDA's food pyramid, are bad for you. Grains turn to sugar almost as quickly as pure sugar turns to sugar. Yes, the fiber is okay for you, but the heavy fiber recommendations that have been touted for the past many years is nothing but laxative-maker income. You'll get plenty of fiber through vegetables and nuts.

Fruit actually turns to sugar in your blood stream more quickly than grains and the FDA has said you need lots of fruit, almost as much as grains, in your daily diet. Sugar piles up on top of sugar.

I'm a huge fan of vegetables, but not all vegetables are created equally. Starches such as corn and potatoes are horrible because they turn to sugar rapidly inside your body. But eat as many colorful, non-starch vegetables that you want. Your hips will shrink and your brain will appreciate it.

At least the FDA didn't put meat on the very *top* of the food pyramid, but they want you to eat far less meat and milk and cheese than sugar in the form of grains, fruits, and indiscriminate vegetables. And fat… such as nuts and olive oil? The worse offender they say. So the FDA puts the fats on the very top.

Fat makes you fat right?

Wrong. You know the answer to that already. Good, healthy fats such as grass-fed butter and organic extra virgin coconut oil don't add size to your waist. It's quite the opposite.

Did you know your brain is composed mostly of fat?

Your brain *requires* fat to be healthy.

You have two choices:

1. Make your brain fat with non-nutritional sugar from grains and lots and lots of fruits and starchy vegetables, or
2. Supply your brain with healthy fats that don't add pounds by eating healthy meats, good dairy, and get plenty of fats from nuts and oils such as coconut, flaxseed, and olive oils.

Your family's blood screenings, which you should consider getting annually, should show the direct results of eating extremely little grain except as a "treat" once in a while, far more fibrous vegetables than fruits, little to no fruit juice, a vast amount of cage-free organic eggs, grass-fed beef, free-range chickens, wild Alaskan salmon, nuts, seeds, olive oil, macadamia nut oil, flaxseed, coconut, and other healthy fats that our brains soak up and utilize like a sponge.

In 1982, the American Heart Association, the American Medical Association, and the USDA issued a dire and, unfortunately, very public warning against fat in food. This is why after only a couple of years it seemed as though every product on the supermarket shelves was sold in a "fat free" version. The public's health has degraded ever since as a direct result.

It's not the fat in foods!

It must be something else and there are only two options left: protein or carbohydrates. All those sugars with non-sugary names aren't made from protein; those are carbohydrates. It's the carbs making us fat and squeezing far more fat matter into our brains where we function far less effectively resulting in our brains being hampered from keeping us fit and trim.

We need to feed our brains and stop feeding ourselves on lies that have *no* basis in fact. But today we can't get all of our brain's needed nutrition from food alone. So many of those "in the know" use supplements, and so should you.

We're getting to all those specifics. Hang on as best you can.

10

THE FANTASTIC 4

With a working knowledge of four *fantastic* neurotransmitters for your body, your brain will be better.

Dopamine – The Reward Chemical

Dopamine is a neurotransmitter that helps transmit signals from your neurons to cells via a synapse.

In plain English? That means that dopamine helps your brain's electrical impulses function smoothly.

Remember that your brain communicates through electrical impulses. When you feel pleasure it's because dopamine is regulating your emotion. Somehow when something pleasurable occurs, or when your brain senses that something might be pleasurable (not necessarily good for you), dopamine is released to cause you to feel the pleasure. Your brain turns on the pleasure switch in a manner of speaking by releasing dopamine.

Dopamine can make us feel pleasure (and reward) and also your brain's release of dopamine encourages you to seek pleasure or take action that might increase pleasure that is close by. It's an amazing thing.

Maybe Dopamine's Why They Call it Dope!

Addictions often come about because of a low amount of dopamine in someone's system. They have a tendency to lack feelings of pleasure and reward due to a lack of dopamine so they seek pleasure and reward where they can find it. A substitute can be found in the short-run through drugs, both prescription, as well as "recreational" drugs.

The problem is that your brain has a tremendous capacity to regulate itself when all four of your nutrient chemicals are in balance. In a healthy brain you will get the right amount of dopamine flowing when you need it and it stops when it's appropriate. But if the brain/body connection goes out of balance and dopamine gets too low, you'll not be able to get enough of the pleasure sensation through normal means so you search elsewhere. And elsewhere is where trouble can begin and addictions can start.

The best thing about dopamine (and your other brain nutrients) is that in the vast majority of people, getting them in balance is much easier than getting off drug addictions. It's far easier (and cheaper!) (and healthier!) to raise your dopamine levels through eating right and supplements than to seek a replacement for low dopamine effects.

How Do I Know if I Have a Dopamine Deficiency?

If you have weight problems you should always suspect low dopamine levels. Also, if you crave excess alcohol and drugs you should suspect low dopamine levels. If you simply don't feel great most of the time you should suspect low dopamine levels.

We gain weight when we over-eat the wrong foods consistently. The weight gain is a result of the overeating and eating bad foods, but the *cause* of the weight gain is almost always found in the brain.

Dopamine is often low when we don't feel satisfied after a meal that seems to satisfy others around us. When we are angry, more often than we should be, our body and emotions are responding to a lack of pleasure and reward that we would otherwise get through a normal production of dopamine.

> **Note:** I will say this elsewhere because of its importance for you. For all of these brain nutrients, a thorough blood test covering your nutritional state as well as other characteristics such as your hormone levels and thyroid and kidney functions is one of the best starting points to determine where you now stand and what you need to work on. If you immediately begin taking the supplements and eating the foods recommended in this book, your brain's good nutritious chemicals will increase. But having a starting point to know which chemical might be at a critically low level means you can attack the worst problem first, and perhaps that alone is going to put you in balance. Yes, when you get a thorough blood test you truly *can* learn which chemical is out of balance!

We're going to take steps to boost your dopamine levels. If your dopamine is too low, that means that you have been doing something to lower your dopamine. Some people don't make enough dopamine naturally due to some chronic problem or illness, but the vast majority of us with low dopamine levels have low levels because we've taught our brains to produce less dopamine. Often we have taught our brains to reduce dopamine by the bad foods we eat.

Sugary foods that produce high sugar content in our blood stream will lower our brain's production of dopamine. If you've read about low-carb diets, they are accurate in their conclusions, but not always in their cause-and-effect. Too many processed foods and desserts turn our blood into thick sugar water, if I might exaggerate just a tad.

Dopamine levels influence all your cravings. If your cravings are out of control your dopamine level is probably out of balance. In addition to sugars and starches, low dopamine people crave caffeine and other stimulants. They also have a tendency to act cranky. The added caffeine helps promote even more crankiness. The cycle can become vicious. Caffeine has benefits. But major caffeine cravings indicate a dopamine problem.

Many people cannot walk away from starchy and sugary foods overnight. They can, however, increase their dopamine quickly through natural supplements and then over time through food and spices. They then can easily switch off the sugar cravings because their brains are producing the pleasure and reward chemical, dopamine, automatically. The cravings and yes, the possible addiction to the bad, starchy, simple carbohydrates will decrease. That makes dopamine increase even more. This makes us crave the bad things even less than before. This makes eating good foods easier. This increases our dopamine. And the merry-go-round actually becomes merry for a change!

Note: Sure, every once in a while we all binge in some way. A desire to binge on a triple-scoop of Rocky

Road steeped in syrup, whipped cream, and bananas might be a temporary reduction in dopamine levels. Our body waxes and wanes in all sorts of ways and a once-in-a-while binge is not a big red flag. A binge of more than once a week, however, is a sure sign of a problem somewhere and dopamine is one of the best places to start looking.

By the way, keep in mind how all this works. Increasing low dopamine levels does not mean you replace your dopamine. Instead, you give your brain the right nutrients to *create* dopamine at healthy levels.

Dopamine for the Rest of Us

For most of us here, dopamine is the primary key nutritional brain chemical. Your metabolism is closely linked to dopamine. That means that if your dopamine is at a good level, then your body becomes an efficient food-burning machine. Your body will tend to store less fat and use food for fuel. To help matters, you will crave fewer foods that cause problems (sugars, grains, and such).

You don't go on a diet to lose weight. You don't exercise to change your metabolism. All of the things we've tried for decades don't work because they're not starting with our brains! If we can get dopamine in balance, with the other brain chemicals, we can get our metabolism in balance, we get our cravings in balance, we appreciate foods that are better for us, and we start looking and feeling great.

Control dopamine and you control your weight.

As you increase your dopamine you'll find an almost instant ability to stay focused on tasks. Higher dopamine levels keep us focused. Your memory, attention span, and ability to learn new things are all affected by dopamine levels. Whenever you eat right, your dopamine levels increase, which will make you feel good and satisfied.

Note: You can raise your dopamine levels somewhat without food, supplements, or drugs by simply relaxing. The best way to do this is take a proactive role in reducing stress that is affecting your life right now. Other good side effects will result too, including a lowered production of adrenaline and a better frame of mind.

Serious Low Dopamine Problems

Weight gain and feeling cranky or depressed are some of the *better* side effects of low dopamine levels. Serious health problems can arise from low dopamine. Not only do some people have problems of addictions due to low dopamine levels, but low dopamine levels have also been linked in serious ways to Parkinson's disease, mental retardation, bipolar disorders, schizophrenia, and other major problems.

If you are overweight and that prompted you to get this book, if you only want to fix your dopamine to lose weight, I'll be happy for you as a bug in a rug. But there's a chance that you'll ward off far more serious problems in the long run too... and that is especially good for you.

An Interesting Side Effect of Low Dopamine

If you've done everything else right to lose weight – reduced simple carbs and exercised more – but you've failed to lose weight (and perhaps even gained weight), you might very well be producing an extremely low amount of dopamine. In these extreme cases you must supplement to get your brain in balance as quickly as possible so that your brain can begin ramping up your metabolism to help you lose weight.

Increase dopamine and you increase your metabolism.

If That Doesn't Convince You, Maybe This Will

You're probably ready to begin boosting your dopamine levels right now. I just caution you about jumping off the deep end because one or more of the other three brain nutrient chemicals might also be low and you should understand how they all work and interact before focusing just on one, no matter how major dopamine is.

But here are a few more nuggets about dopamine before we move to the others.

The number of dopamine receptors in your brain decreases as you gain more and more weight. The amount of fat you carry is dis-proportional to your dopamine receptors. With fewer receptors your brain will not get the "I'm happy, satisfied, and full" signal as intensely, which causes you to overindulge more.

> **Note:** It's the hormone called *leptin* that tells us when we're full. Simple carbohydrates mask our leptin production so we don't know when we are full. Our leptin is broken. Fortunately, a healthy diet along with supplementation will quickly repair leptin levels.

Some personality problems arise due to low dopamine including: eccentricity, shy loner syndrome (introversion), procrastination, masochism and aggression, codependency, and obsessive-compulsiveness. Low dopamine levels are often implicated in ADHD diagnosis.

I cannot stress it enough: low dopamine equals big (or more) belly fat.

> **Note:** One reason for this is that for every one of your brain chemicals that is deficient, a hormone takes its place. Cortisol takes the place of dopamine. When stressed you naturally burn more dopamine. Cortisol is considered the "obesity hormone." Cortisol forces your metabolism to slow down.

Low dopamine levels make you feel as though you have no fire. You need a stimulant like coffee to get going it seems (hopefully you choose a 10-Hour Coffee Diet coffee). Fortunately, the more dopamine your brain produces, the faster your metabolism gets.

Listen up! Here's the Real Reason Why You Want More Dopamine: Higher dopamine levels improve your sex drive.

Serotonin – The Happy Chemical

Want to be happy? Increase your serotonin!

Serotonin improves your mood, helps you sleep better, and makes you more even-tempered.

Do you know how good you feel after a big Thanksgiving turkey dinner? You just want to go to sleep. And you probably have heard that it's the tryptophan in turkey that does that. L-tryptophan is an amino acid that comes in turkey and some other foods. When that food begins to break down, the L-tryptophan amino acid gets converted to an even longer, more expensive-sounding term called 5-Hydroxytrytophan. And it's that 5-Hydroxytrytophan that converts to serotonin and goes straight to your brain.

In normal language, it means this: Eat turkey and feel good enough to relax and go to sleep. Serotonin makes you feel good, happy, relaxed, and gives you that "all is right with the world" attitude.

> **Note:** Honesty is the best policy, right? I'd be remiss if I blamed your sleepiness *just* on the turkey. When you eat a *lot* for a Thanksgiving meal, and who doesn't, your body is going to want to slow you down to have more energy to digest all that food. The sleepiness you get after any big meal is a direct result of your body saying, "I can't digest all this food *and* keep you active, so slow down!" But think back to how you felt last Thanksgiving after turkey. It was different from the typical huge meal after-effect. Yes, you feel incredibly stuffed (almost like a stuffed turkey, right?) but there's not the typical "I can't believe I ate the *whooole* thing!" feeling. It's a far more relaxing and feel-good feeling than just "I'm too full." That extra-good feeling of being full comes from your brain's serotonin kicking into high gear thanks to the turkey's tryptophan and 5-Hydroxytrytophan.

Serotonin allows you to experience pleasure and feel good about yourself. You feel alive. Without serotonin we don't feel much of anything. Cravings increase that are usually not good. Low serotonin levels result in an increased salt craving for example. Salt is one of the maligned foods of the past 50 years and is far less deadly than it's been blamed for. Still, a craving for salt can result in a salt/potassium imbalance that does eventually cause you problems. A repaired serotonin level can help repair your salt craving and help return your sodium/potassium levels back to where they should be: in balance.

How Do I Know if I Have a Serotonin Deficiency?

Diet and serotonin go hand in hand as you just saw with the turkey. Other foods and supplements affect our serotonin levels due to various nutrients or nutrient deficiencies in our foods.

The bottom line of a low level of serotonin is a feel-bad state of mind and body. You just want to give up. You have low self-esteem and you often worry too much about tiny things. That worry can easily turn into irrational fear and anxiety that becomes long-term phobias. For women, PMS is more severe and for men (in general) anger and aggression can become a problem. Women need more serotonin during menstruation.

Note: You might recall that aggression is possible from a lack of dopamine also, which is why you don't want to diagnose yourself yet and just start fixing one of these brain nutritional chemicals. You need to know the whole picture and fix the whole picture. If you're low on more than one of the brain chemicals, then a general routine of supplements and food that boosts all of them will help them go into alignment. You won't overdose on one that you happen not to be deficient in right now. Your brain is a great regulator. It's only when you use drugs as the "solution" that you introduce a danger of overdosing on one or more of the chemicals and having to deal with that. You brain won't be able to regulate high states of chemicals injected/snorted/smoked through drugs if you don't magically happen onto the exact dosage required each time you take your drugs.

Sleep will turn into restless sleep that will turn into insomnia in many people with low serotonin levels. Your ability to move forward mentally when at work will be hampered also; you'll have trouble moving onto new thoughts and therefore new projects because you'll find yourself returning to current and past work repeatedly.

As with dopamine, serotonin deficiencies can become circular and you'll cause your serotonin levels to decrease if you don't recognize the problem and work to reverse your serotonin deficiencies now. Stress, for example, is a major serotonin robber and the fears and anxiety that comes with low serotonin levels add to your stress, thus reducing your serotonin levels further.

Serotonin-deficient people can become suspicious and self-absorbed. This leads to wanting to be alone more. This leads to eating worse through so-called comfort foods and junk foods (which are often the same foods). This bad diet leads to lesser levels of serotonin and the cycle just gets worse due to the downward spiral we unwittingly put ourselves into.

Your insulin regulation is partially controlled by your serotonin levels as well. You'll crave sugars and starches more than usual. You could develop an insulin resistance, which is something to avoid if possible.

Note: Are you finding that the symptoms for low serotonin *and* the symptoms for low dopamine way too familiar to you? Many people have low levels of some or all the brain nutrient chemicals. It's difficult and often impossible to determine the specific chemical you're lowest in because so many symptoms overlap. Don't be surprised if tests show that you're deficient in more than one.

Low serotonin induced anxiety levels can cause people to seek psychiatric help. Getting antidepressants will only shield the true problem by masking it. Antidepressants, if they work for you, are keeping your anxiety down but you're not solving the root problem. And it turns out that you may be working against the very problem because the overuse of antidepressants – guess what – actually can reduce serotonin even further.

Although low serotonin levels can be the result of a genetic disorder, as can any of the Fantastic Four primary brain nutrient chemicals, in almost every case a low level is the result of a bad diet and bad health patterns. If an antidepressant doesn't damage your health more, it often does nothing but cost you money. Obviously severe cases are the exception, but we're dealing with the norm. You'll soon see that supplements such as St. John's Wort, walking around your home or down the block a few times, getting some sun, and perhaps even taking up a new hobby does wonders for most of us who experience the blahs.

Low Serotonin Clues

One way that low serotonin reveals itself as deficient is simple: you crave salty foods such as potato chips and or refined carbohydrates such as pasta and bread. This is your body's attempt to boost energy levels by turning on those cravings.

Unfortunately, giving in to those cravings will reduce serotonin and make you quickly plummet to new energy lows.

Ways to Increase Serotonin

You surely know by now that I'm going to tell you that you can increase your serotonin through supplementation and diet. That is true and that certainly is the approach I'd use. Prescription drugs can work, but why mess with their expense and risk when you don't have to?

Plus, serotonin is special in that you can boost it in other ways too. One way is to get more sun!

Let the Sunshine In!

Our solar system's good old sun has gotten a bad rap for about four decades now and it's time to turn the tide around. Just like the lie that "fat makes you fat," one of the biggest lies in recent history is that sun exposure is bad for us.

The sun is *good for you.* And to really make things bad for those who have said otherwise, there is actually talk now about putting warning labels on *sunscreen lotions* to warn against possible cancer-causing properties of their use. The sun does not seem to give us skin cancer in spite of the old wives' tales to the contrary. In fact it's not just the sunscreen lotion itself that is said to possibly be the culprit of the increased skin-related cancers over the past three or four decades, but it's their *intended use* that has caused that increase; that keeping the healthy sun off our bodies invites more skin cancer problems.

> **Note:** Too much sun, meaning day after day of high exposure with no attempt to cover our flesh will burn us and that excess will ruin our skin, the largest organ of our bodies. But that is not what we're talking about. Even a typical day at the beach, once or twice a week, *without* the dangerous sunscreen lotions, is doing hardly anything more than giving us a healthy dose of sun.

Vitamin D3 deficiencies have been so great the past few decades that finally even the mainstream media sources and mainstream health sources have begun discussing the dangers of its drastically low levels. Vitamin D3 is known as the "sun's vitamin" precisely because we get vitamin D3 from the sun's exposure. We can get far more sun than we've been told, but it turns out we only need about 20 minutes of sun exposure daily to get ample vitamin D3. But not all of us live in areas where the sun shines daily. Fortunately, quality sources of D3 supplementation are available.

D3 doesn't work alone. One of the biggest benefits of D3 is that it is a catalyst for helping calcium work effectively in our bodies. If you take calcium supplements and drink lots of good, raw, whole, healthy milk and eat great sources of beef and chicken and eggs, far less of that great calcium will work for you if you don't also get enough D3. I take 5,000 to 10,000 IUs of D3 daily depending on the time of year and how active I plan to be outside.

But this book isn't about D3, although I sure hope you get enough D3. D3 is *so* critical to our health that it was worth a detour to tell you the above. I'd suggest that putting D3 as a priority equal to that of the brain chemicals themselves. But speaking of those, let's get back to serotonin. In addition to D3, guess what the sun also boosts in our bodies? Yep, serotonin. You'll not only boost your serotonin through diet and supplementation, but you should also go play outside more.

You'll do your brain and your body good!

GABA – The Excitement Chemical

Can you say gamma-aminobutyric acid?

Yea, I can't either. I'm glad it's also called *GABA*.

GABA is the brain nutrient chemical that controls your excitability by regulating your nervous system. Our production of GABA controls how excitable our response to life's stimuli is. And GABA is also responsible for regulating other factors of our health, most notably for our purposes: our muscle tone.

In addition to the muscle tone controller, the excitability factor of GABA can't be ignored for weight loss purposes either. The reverse effect of GABA's excitement regulation is that GABA also controls our calmness. When we're calm and assured, we are confident and have far better control over our lives, our eating habits, our enjoyment of life, and our overall success at whatever we do. Once again, it's our brains that control our bodies and control our success or failure at activities such as dieting.

How Do I Know if I Have a GABA Deficiency?

GABA, being an excitability controller, is also responsible for controlling anxiety (you might recall that serotonin does this too). Anxiety may very well be a sign of a GABA imbalance and low serotonin too. If your GABA goes out of balance in the other direction, it can have difficulty regulating your calming factors as well as making you feel far more depressed than you should under normal circumstances. In this case, GABA is regulating your mood down too much.

This extreme mood swing ability leads to some serious lifestyle problems, not unlike some of the problems associated with the other brain chemicals:

- Alcoholism
- Depression
- Panic attacks
- Bipolar maladies

Note: These can go hand-in-hand. An imbalance of GABA leading to over-calmness so great that depression results can very well lead to alcoholism for example.

Are you getting the message that these four brain chemicals are vital for your health and well-being? Your body won't be in balance until these are in balance. You won't feel good until these are in balance. You won't lose weight until you begin boosting your mind's nutrients. I don't call them the Fantastic Four for nothing.

When your brain functions improperly, due to a bad diet, lack of nutrients, and even stress, your brain's GABA receptor stops adding GABA to your system. These and other factors can decrease the ability of your brain's GABA to function properly and in the correct quantities.

Sometimes genetics plays a role in improper GABA production, but like the other brain chemicals, genetics is a far less-common cause. Diet and stress are typically the most common factors that affect GABA.

Increased GABA Advantages

My goal in this section of the 10-Hour Coffee Diet book is to express the importance of a balanced brain over weight loss. But weight loss for those who have problems in that area is critical too, because obesity brings all sorts of problems onto a person who otherwise wouldn't have them.

It's also my hope that you don't just focus on your weight when you look in the mirror. You can be thin and look unhealthy... and *be* unhealthy. I want you to be the best you can be and that means getting all the physical and emotional baggage out of the way so you can focus on what is important: your well-being, and that means more than what the scale says.

The fact that GABA helps you maintain muscle tone is a wonderful reason to put your brain's GABA in balance, but so much more is tied to GABA too. So many problems can begin to be helped. As you increase your GABA production, the following problems will likely lessen also:

- Alcohol withdrawal symptoms
- Anxiety
- Schizophrenia
- High blood pressure
- Increased effect of insulin for diabetics
- Suppressed appetite (!)

- Reduced PMS symptoms
- Reversal of some forms of depression[52]

The GABA-Pain Connection

Dr. Eric Braverman, M.D., writes a lot about the brain chemicals. He describes how chronic pain can cause people to eat more. I would assume this is the result of needing comfort from the pain. Comfort foods typically come to mind for the solution to being uncomfortable.

Comfort foods are misnamed. Traditional comfort foods like potatoes and corn do *not* comfort your body, but instead simply add starchy carbs that affect your body negatively. Comfort foods only temporarily solve a sugar craving that we often get when we get improper signals that cause a need for reward or calmness or energy. Comfort foods will give us short-term relief from chronic pain by causing us to forget it for a while. The problem is that such food will do long-term damage to our bodies and mind so a vicious cycle results. And of course, junk food of all kinds tends to temporarily satisfy a short-term need for comfort at the expense of long-term problems.

Overeating maladies such as binging and wanting to "try one of everything at the buffet" is typically connected to GABA problems. Dr. Braverman describes how low-GABA people are unable to set boundaries. The fact that chronic pain somehow encourages us to seek comfort foods and this inability to set eating boundaries multiples bad eating behaviors further.

It doesn't do our chronic pain any good either. Dr. Braverman describes how chronic pain can drain your GABA, but he also describes that low GABA can create and encourage forms of chronic pain. So either GABA is a source of the pain or a reason your pain is still there. Either way, you want more GABA production!

GABA Monitors the Other Three

GABA is not considered the most important of the four chemicals for most people. GABA doesn't show itself in symptoms as readily as deficiencies in dopamine and serotonin. Those two chemicals often are culprits with the majority of brain/body problems it seems.

Still, there is another primary reason why you should never ignore your GABA levels and why you should focus on boosting GABA through supplementation and diet as well as the others: GABA helps control and regulate all your other brain chemicals.

In other words, your dopamine *can* be out of whack because your GABA is out of whack.

Consider this: GABA is opposite of dopamine and acetylcholine (you'll read about that next). GABA and serotonin create calm and order. Also, too much stress from not getting enough sleep due to not enough GABA burns out your dopamine, acetylcholine, and serotonin. The connection to GABA as the monitor of the other three cannot be stressed enough. Even though a deficiency in GABA might not show itself as fully as a deficiency in the others, if one or more of the others are out of balance a lack of GABA may very well be one of the major contributors.

Acetylcholine – The Nervy Chemical

Acetylcholine is a nervous system-controlling chemical. Acetylcholine regulates both your peripheral nervous system (nerves outside your brain and spinal cord) and your central nervous system.

Being a nervous system chemical means that our memories are affected by our acetylcholine production. Elderly patients who experience short-term memory loss often are found with low levels of acetylcholine because acetylcholine tends to decrease as we age. This age-related memory lapse is a common and normal function, due in part to a decreased acetylcholine production, and shouldn't always be associated with Alzheimer's Disease which is a far more serious and unnatural brain disorder that primarily affects some elderly but can occur at young ages too. Still, Alzheimer Disease patients are often found with an acetylcholine decrease of up to 90% of normal... so Alzheimer's connection to low acetylcholine cannot be stressed enough.

How Do I Know if I Have An Acetylcholine Deficiency?

Obviously, if you have memory troubles you should suspect acetylcholine as a possible cause.

But acetylcholine works to do much more than help your memory. Given its importance in your nervous system it acts like oil in a gearbox, making connections work better and faster and more efficiently. Those connections are in your brain, your spine, and in your muscles too!

Low acetylcholine means your body responds more slowly. Your wheels aren't greased well in other words. If your body responds more slowly to stimuli and thoughts and ideas, by now you should be able to guess why: your *brain* is responding more slowly. As your brain goes, your body goes.

An acetylcholine deficiency causes you to be forgetful and makes you mentally and physically slower. The lubrication and insulation that acetylcholine provides for your brain (and muscles) shows up in the form of fat, and not quality healthy fat that you need, but an over-abundance of fat cells inside where there should be fewer fat cells. Deficiencies in acetylcholine make you crave the bad, deep-fried, potato-based, sugary and starchy kinds of fatty foods that you should avoid like the plague.

In other words, what you need most to avoid is what you will crave the most.

One of the most obvious signs of acetylcholine deficiency is a big craving for fatty foods because of the loss of good acetylcholine-based fat.

Some people's memory lapse, due to low acetylcholine, shows itself as a weight management problem. People literally forgot that they recently ate. So they will eat sooner than they otherwise might eat, thus adding extra calories when your body is still processing the previous meal's calories.

Your brain's connections are insulated in the way electrical wires are insulated. The insulation is called *myelin.* Myelin consists of fat and protein. Multiple Sclerosis (MS) patients have an erosion of their myelin, which is caused by a body's natural immune system attacking the myelin by mistake... causing *demyelination.* The nerves then function poorly, not unlike electrical wires that short circuit and carry current poorly when their insulation is removed.[53]

Being overweight decreases your acetylcholine or at least decreases your acetylcholine's effectiveness. Your nerves don't have the freedom and room to function well with fat slowing them down. In spite of the fact that your myelin is composed of fat (and protein), excess brain fat hampers and does not help your nervous system's connections.

A deficiency in acetylcholine can cause some internal problems that are even worse than the other three brain chemical deficiencies. Your nervous system's balance is crucial. And to feel good and have muscle tone and sexy curves that others will envy you must balance acetylcholine!

Bladder and Libido Issues Too

Still more is on the line with acetylcholine.

Your bladder and bowels can begin to misbehave. By not eliminating waste efficiently, toxins build in your body and cause more problems. The more problems your body has to battle the fewer resources it has to get you balanced and feeling great. And the worse you feel, the less you want to do to reverse that feeling.

Speaking of feeling bad... sexual dysfunction can occur with low levels of acetylcholine production too. This simply reinforces your emotional downer state and causes relationship problems also. This causes you to avoid interacting with the people closest to you, which further reduces your ability to move forward and get back into balance.

Increased Acetylcholine Advantages

When you balance your acetylcholine your nervous system has a chance to function properly once again. Your entire body begins to reverse the negative course it's on due to low levels of acetylcholine. Being that your central nervous system, your brain/spinal connection, is affected by acetylcholine, so many hidden problems can begin to reverse themselves as you increase your body's acetylcholine.

The first thing you or others may notice as you increase acetylcholine is that your cognitive abilities become sharper. Your brain has to waste fewer resources on body battles so it is freed up for critical thinking skills and problem solving. Your approach, therefore, to every problem and challenge in life will improve. That means your ability and desire to avoid bad foods that cause you harm while seeking foods that make you feel even better grows. Your willpower increases not just for good foods but also for companionship.

Your muscle tone has a better chance to develop as you feel better again. You'll more likely feel good enough to exercise and eat foods that build your body instead of the badly named "comfort foods" that have been tearing you down. You will stop forgetting to eat so you won't feel starvation pangs that tend to make you binge. You also stop forgetting that you just ate and are eating again. Basically, you just plain stop forgetting.

As you age, your ability to ward off normal memory lapses and abnormal memory problems such as Alzheimer's will increase by having healthy acetylcholine levels. Your chance at a much fuller life lengthens. Your chance at a longer life lengthens also because diabetes and other age-shortening problems will decrease. This all occurs because the signals in your brain, insulated by the myelin, connect better, communicate faster, and function more effectively.

Are You Up to the Challenge?

You might find it intriguing to learn that you can increase your acetylcholine by reading a lot and challenging yourself somewhat beyond your mental and physical comfort zone. Our bodies are amazing machines that strive in every way to return to normal balance all the time in spite of what we do to them. In challenging yourself, your brain will more easily see low amounts of acetylcholine and will do its best to produce more.

This is hard to do, no doubt. Low acetylcholine means that last thing you'll want to do, and sometimes you won't even have the memory to remember to do so, is challenge yourself more. But just like our muscles that grow bigger and better as we tear them down through healthy exercise, our brains will do their best to provide chemicals we need as we challenge our brains.

Watch more *Jeopardy* and read more books. With your brain in balance, you will accelerate your ability to lose weight and get healthier through other diet and exercise advice, tips, and tricks.

Keep this in mind as you begin to re-balance your brain, your body, and your life. Take an extra challenge or two that you might have avoided. It can be simple such as trying to single-handedly solve a problem at work that is assigned to several on your team. Grab a book and read it outside on a sunny day, stacking the wonderful vitamin D3-producing sun rays with your brain challenge while eating a delicious organic lunch you brought from home with spices that make it taste as though you bought it in the most expensive 5-star restaurant in Paris!

How can you make food like that? Glad you asked, just use the kinds of foods, spices, oils, and drinks that build better brains. Turn the page to see all about that.

11

FOODS THAT NOURISH, REVITALIZE, AND ENERGIZE YOUR BRAIN

Previously, we focused on what the brain nutrient chemicals were all about. It's not just about weight loss, but lasting weight loss *and good* health that you can achieve. You need to deal with the Fantastic Four, the four brain chemicals:

- Dopamine
- Serotonin
- GABA
- Acetylcholine

Fix the brain first. Your body will follow.

Let's get started on doing just that.

The Food Approach

A great way to attack your brain's lack of nutrients is with diet and you should begin immediately. Determine which brain chemicals you need to work on most, and possibly even better, get a blood test to be sure of where you stand not only on your brain nutrients, but other important body aspects such as blood sugar, hormones, iodine, kidney functions, and everything else you can talk your doctor into testing. Why wouldn't you want a baseline to know where you stand today and what your body needs to get it running at its optimal performance?

Note: Notice I mentioned iodine. You need to make sure that any blood test you get includes your thyroid-related health stats. I believe that in general, iodine deficiency is second only to our D3 deficiency in the modern world. The required amount of iodine is probably so low as to be laughable if it were not so dangerous. Many people are put on thyroid medicine that would otherwise benefit from a short time on iodine supplements. You may need to take up to 30 mgs of iodine tablets in supplement form just to get up to normal, healthy levels. But the FDA's daily requirements are not stated in mg's but in mcg's, from 110 mcg to 290 mcg daily. That means they suggest you get *micrograms* of iodine when what you probably need are *milligrams*; in other words move the decimal point to the right... meaning that the daily requirements are possibly 100 times too low for us today!

The reason you want to approach brain repair through food is because:

1. You need to eat anyway.
2. Food that fixes your brain seems to help many other health problems also.
3. Food that fixes your brain seems to ward off common health problems in your future.
4. Food that fixes your brain seems to make you thinner and improve your muscle tone.
5. Food that fixes your brain seems to turn on cravings for *more* of the same good food and less of the bad stuff that damages your brain and body.
6. Food that fixes your brain is what people ate for thousands of years. The past 35-45 years of bad dietary advice can't reverse the good that good foods do no matter how much the advocates of bad food try to promote it.

Here's the thing. Tons of diets and eating suggestions exist. They fall into camps such as:

- Low fat, low protein
- High fat, low protein
- High carb, low protein, low fat
- High carb, high fat
- No carb, high fat, medium protein
- And everything else you can think of

The reason food falls into three primary categories of carbohydrate, fat, and protein is because food literally *does* exist in those three states. Food impacts your body through the type of food it is.

How can one group say that a low-carb, high protein diet will cause you to lose weight while another says that only a high-carb, low protein diet will cause you to lose weight?

Pretty much any kind of diet can help you to lose weight immediately. Many of the diets that would cause you to gain weight under their approaches make it so you temporarily lose weight because they restrict your caloric levels so severely that you don't get enough calories to gain weight (or to survive for very long by the way).

It is possible to lose weight, at least for a short time, under just about any combination of food advice.

The Two Primary Battlegrounds

In spite of tons of diets around, diet suggestions most typically fall into two opposing camps:

- High-carb, low fat, low protein
- Low-carb, high fat, medium-to-high protein

I can save us both a bunch of time. Your brain prefers the second way of eating. So does your body. Fortunately, this is the way you will eat when you follow the 10-Hour Coffee Diet plan.

All four brain chemical nutrients benefit from and are boosted more when you eat a low-carb diet that is rich in proteins and healthy fats.

The Carbs in "Low Carb"

The carbohydrates that you eat in brain-healthy, low-carb diets are leafy, fibrous, green vegetables like spinach, cabbage, chard, and kale. Eating those in their raw form is fine. Cooking them is fine too, but don't overcook them because their vitamins start breaking down as soon as you begin cooking them.

Colorful vegetables are also part of any brain-healthy diet. Beets, carrots, green and red and yellow peppers, squash, all those kinds of veggies are ones that make salads look good and that make your brain feel good.

Low-carb never means no-carb.

The Protein

Always let your taste and bank account guide you when they must, but begin making an effort to improve the quality of the protein you feed yourself and your family.

The protein you need most is a good quality animal protein. That means organic, if possible, but more important than organic is that your beef is grass-fed (locally raised if possible), your chickens are grown cage-free where they don't live from cradle-to-grave in their own excrement in a chicken house in Arkansas, where your milk is raw if you can source such a place,[54] and the pork you eat (if you want to) comes from happy pigs who wallow in fields and streams on the farms where they are raised. See the movie *Food, Inc.*, if you think my suggestions here are a little extreme.

I highly suggest a book by Dr. William Campbell called *The Truth about Raw Milk.*

If you want to look into this further, the Weston Price organization will let you know if you have any raw milk sources close to where you live. Raw milk: it does a body and brain good! One thing I want to note right here. As much as I love raw milk, I don't want you to use it in your 10-Hour Coffee Diet coffees. Use unsweetened almond milk.

The Fats in High Fat Diets

Your brain is mostly fat. Guess what you need to make sure your diet has in it? Fat!

The brain fats you need don't come from whole ice cream and Snickers bars. The fat you need comes in the form of good oils such as olive oil, coconut oil, grass-fed butter, flaxseed oils, seeds, nuts, fish oil, cod liver oil, and the fat in meats.

If you don't know the source of your meat, then it's almost for certain bad for you. In other words, you almost certainly are eating beef raised on nothing but corn grain its whole life instead of grass that it was designed to be raised on. You are eating cows that would be sick and would have died long before they were slaughtered if they weren't pumped full of antibiotics from birth.

Yech!

The problem with fat in such meat is that the toxins *always* travel to the fat. If you eat unhealthy beef, as you certainly do with all that is USDA certified and in most restaurants, then you should trim all excess fat and get as lean of cuts as possible. The toxins are not worth the fat. But this means you don't get good animal fat where you should be getting them.

So, it's *best* to know the source of most meat you eat. Eating grass-fed, hormone-free beef and pork as well as cage-free chickens means the fat in those meats are wonderful for your body and your brains and you need the fat.

If you don't want to get fat from eating fat then you should eat more fat! As Gary Taubes shows scientifically at the cell level, eating healthy animal fat makes you lean and makes your mind happy.

Yes that's right, fat helps you get lean in spite of the "typical advice."

The Brain's Favorite Food Fundamentals Skinned, Boiled, and Presented in a Nutshell

Avoid any and all simple carbs.

This means sugar. This means pasta. This means bread in excess of a slice or *maybe* two every few days and that slice needs to be loaded with nuts and best made from scratch using organic, raw wheat that you grind into flour right before baking your bread. Sound like too much work? Then skip the bread. But don't eat most bread, including "whole wheat" bread. Bread, in general, is one step away from sugar in your body.

Avoiding all simple carbs also means avoiding all those corn and potato chips. Yea, they taste great, but they are one step away from sugar as far as your body is concerned.

> **Note:** Have you ever wondered why many restaurants bring a breadbasket before every meal? Even worse, have you ever wondered why many Mexican restaurants make sure there's a big basket of chips on your table *before you even see a menu?* Simple carbs make you hungry... and bread and chips are superb at making you *real* hungry! Eating lots of chips before you look at a menu actually ramps up your craving switches causing you to want more than you would have wanted without the chips or bread. Our brains know this, which is why they react so badly to simple carbs and sugars. But, our stomachs and tongues aren't as smart as the gray matter between our ears.

Bottom line? Avoid corn and potatoes. These are starchy vegetables and, do I need to say it, they are one step away from sugar.

(I'm assuming I don't have to tell you to avoid desserts as much as possible. I know I'm no fun. But I want your brains to function at their peak performance. Treat desserts as special occasions.

Your Brain Chemicals' Favorite Foods

In general, a low-carb, high-quality animal protein, raw whole dairy and eggs (eat the whole egg and don't overcook them; poached and over-easy are the best preparation methods and make sure you get eggs from cage-free hens), and lots of quality fats will boost every single brain chemical. Fortunately, even Wal-Mart now sells eggs that come from healthy, free-range chickens. Eating healthy is easier than ever before.

Your brain's Fantastic Four chemical nutrients will be as powerful as the *Fantastic Four* heroes in Marvel comic books if you eat right.

As a general rule, eliminate all simple carbs from your life, source your meat and dairy from the healthiest places available to you, and get good fats in organic seeds, nuts, and good oils (we'll cover fats more in the next chapter).

Still, each brain chemical does prefer a specific sub-group of those kinds of foods. Let's look at each of your brain chemical's favorite foods.

Dopamine and Food

Sugar depletes dopamine. No surprise there, especially after the previous sections right?

Switch to Stevia whenever possible if you must sweeten tea or coffee or something else.

What kinds of foods do your brain's dopamine receptors enjoy most and function best with? Primarily you must keep this in mind when trying to improve dopamine: protein is the building block for creating dopamine. Many foods are rich in protein. High-carb promoters completely are in the dark about the benefits of protein-rich foods including:

- Animal proteins like beef, turkey, and chicken
- Dairy in the form of raw, whole milk and cheeses made from raw milk (if you can't get cheese made from raw milk at least buy only organic cheese)
- Kefir and yogurt (real yogurt, not the low-fat kind)

Kefir and yogurt fall into the protein category, but like some special carbohydrate foods such as sauerkraut, miso wine, organic sour cream, and soy sauce, kefir and yogurt are *fermented foods*. These literally are foods that are allowed to sour and ferment before you eat them.

If that sounds gross, every piece of cheese you've ever eaten has probably been fermented during its creation. Real parmesan cheese (not the stuff in the shakers, but the cheese made only in Parma, Italy and imported here called *Parmigiano-Reggiano* cheese) literally sits on a shelf at room temperature *for two years* before it's sold!

Your brain and your body *love* fermented food.

Note: If you just won't or can't make your own yogurt and kefir, get organic Greek yogurt and not the sweet stuff that is just one step from ice cream that you find in the little white cups near the dairy section. They are loaded with sugar (often disguised) and soy (never disguised for some odd reason). *Oikos* Greek yogurt is a good brand that we sometimes use. It comes from Stoneyfield Farms and you can learn more about them in the must-watch movie, *Food, Inc.*

The reason you want fermented foods *daily* is that your gut needs fermented foods. You often get sick in the head from colds and allergies because your *gut* is lacking the flora needed to attack toxins that are always around us. Whereas you fix your brain and you fix your body, if you fix your gut you fix a lot of routine sicknesses that you'd otherwise get. The world around us is unnatural with toxins galore. Our soil and food lacks what it all used to have. Loading up our guts with good bacteria, called *probiotics*, enables our brains to function well and our bodies to ward off sickness, even after direct exposure to sickness.

Dopamine loves yogurt and the other fermented foods. You want more dopamine. Eat fermented foods.

Serotonin and Food

What food does serotonin like?

Serotonin likes much of the same things that dopamine brain receptors like! That makes it easy to boost both when you enjoy:

- Animal proteins like beef, turkey, and chicken
- Dairy in the form of raw, whole milk, grass-fed butter, and cheeses made from raw milk or organic cheese
- Fish

Serotonin is also helped by eating low-carb, fibrous vegetables such as:

- Spinach
- Broccoli
- Oats

Oats are new to the equation. Oats are grains and you should severely limit all grains. Still we never want to toss out the baby with the bath water and if oats help your serotonin levels (dopamine also will benefit from oats some) then don't avoid oats completely. But as always, stack your advantages!

Oatmeal that you get in a box is *not* good for you no matter what the box says. At least it's not as good as it should be for you. When they take the original grain called an *oat groat* and press it to make oats for oatmeal, you have only a few minutes to an hour or two before all of the vitamins are gone from that opened, pressed oat groat kernel. Once it goes into a box, forget about it.

You can buy organic buckets of raw, oat groats from places like Walton Foods (WaltonFeed.com). Get a manual oat grinder and press your own fresh oatmeal a few minutes before you cook and eat your oatmeal. The result is oatmeal that actually contains healthy nutrients… enough to make up for the fact it's a grain.

The same is true of wheat germ. Wheat is healthy and has lots of nutrients. So why do bread manufacturers have to "fortify" bread with vitamins? All the vitamins are gone long before the bread gets to our store shelves. By getting properly packaged wheat germ and by grinding our own organic wheat right before we make bread, those vitamins and minerals are all intact and go into our systems. Nobody who makes bread from scratch at home has to "fortify" it with manufactured vitamins!

One kind of fat that benefits serotonin is fat from an avocado, technically a vegetable, but a wonderful source of fat. Mexican food is wonderful for the brain because as long as you don't eat the tortillas, chips, and rice, all the meat, salsa, vegetables, beans, sour cream, and guacamole you get in Mexican food are all fantastic for your brain. This of course is most true if you locate a Mexican restaurant that understands the importance of organic or grass-fed beef. But, lacking that you can make your own Mexican food and your brain will begin to repair right away *and you'll begin to lose weight!*

Get some avocados and turn them into delicious, fresh guacamole. By the way, avocados *do* stay good in your refrigerator if you eat only half of one and want to save the other. Keep the big seed in the half you save, put it in a baggie, and it'll store nicely in your fridge a few extra days.

> **Note:** Dopamine levels can increase with brown rice just as GABA is influenced in a positive way by corn. Still, there is so much healthier food available that you simply don't have to load your body up with grains like brown rice and corn. Much of the meat you get is corn-fed and you benefit – albeit negatively – from that cow's lifelong diet of corn and you don't ever need one more bite of corn for your body if you can substitute a less starchy vegetable... and you can *always* substitute a less starchy, more leafy vegetable in place of corn and rice.

By the way, you don't see me suggesting many fruits and we'll return to the subject of fruits shortly. But if you're a smoothie lover then you know how bananas can help a smoothie not only taste good, but it adds a nice texture that you might miss if you omit bananas from your diet. (And I suggest you do omit them; bananas are a high-glycemic natural food; they pack on pounds by turning to sugar very fast.) Instead of a banana put half an avocado in your smoothie! It adds a similar texture and actually improves the taste quite a bit if you've got berries and green veggies in the mix, as you almost certainly will have with healthy green smoothies. Trust me, I love bananas. It's hard for me to say to avoid them. At the very least, do what I do and eat them less often.

Dopamine and Your Dinner Time

Dr. Braverman, MD, who has written extensively about brain chemistry, says that the *time* of day that you eat affects serotonin. Eating later at night means that you are less hungry in the daytime. Your body doesn't feel the need to "break its overnight fast" at breakfast. Not only does eating too late affect your morning eating, but it also can give you sleep problems. Dr. Braverman's advice goes hand-in-hand with the 10-Hour Coffee Diet.

This is not universal and if you generally feel as though your serotonin level is adequate, both from a blood test and also by a lack of the serotonin-deficient symptoms mentioned earlier, but you enjoy eating a late dinner, by all means go ahead and do so. Some health advocates buck the trend and suggest that you eat more at night than we're typically told to do. Our stomach's digestion consumes a lot of energy, which is why you feel sleepy after a big lunch. You may want to have your biggest meal for dinner (as recommended in the Traditional 10-Hour Coffee Diet protocol) and begin the process of slowing down for the day (assuming you're not a night shift worker) and you are headed for bed soon where all your body's resources can work on digesting that big meal.

Many people sleep better on a full stomach so don't make serotonin a reason to stop eating late unless you have good reason to believe your serotonin is low. You might try supplements and increase your serotonin-preferred foods before changing your routine of eating late if you want to keep up your current eating schedule as much as possible.

Certainly the people in Italy, Greece, and other Mediterranean areas eat big meals late at night and have been doing so as a culture for centuries without grossly affecting their sleep or serotonin… or weight. Still, if you've tried other ways to boost serotonin and haven't been as successful as you'd like, you should try eating earlier to see if things change for the better then. It's my guess that if you want to maintain a late-night eating routine you'll be able to through supplementation and food choices.

> **Note:** One reason the experts tell us not to eat much later in the day is that we're less active and don't have as much time to work it off. This sounds logical, but there seems to be little evidence we burn our food longer if we eat it earlier. Certainly the Mediterranean countries, that as a whole eat very late, don't have the weight issues as much as we do.

GABA and Food

GABA-building foods fall more into the complex carbohydrate choices and less in the protein and fat categories. You'll get your complex carbs in the form of vegetables. Beans give you a double benefit in that they provide protein as well as a vegetable source of complex carbs.

Some of the GABA-boosting foods are:

- Beans (just about any kind, if you like them, eat them)
- Lentils
- Peas
- Kale
- Broccoli
- Colorful vegetables such as carrots and beets and turnips

Obviously, always buy organic veggies when you can in order to stack your advantages. Otherwise you get unnatural things like pesticides, food colorings, and injections that your body has to fight instead of being able to devote all resources to pulling out the nutrients.

The better place to get vegetables is to open your home's back door and pick them out of your own garden. Let's face it, our busy lives today make that difficult, but if you can, you will boost your complex carbohydrates' brain nutrients so high, it'll be like NASA put a rocket on every cell in your food!

Sourcing of Beans, Lentils, and Peas

You can order 5- and 10-pound buckets of organic, nitrogen-packed beans, lentils, and peas from Walton Foods (WaltonFeed.com) and they stay good and fresh for up to a decade. You'll save *a tremendous* amount of money and have delicious beans ready to go. This is where you can also get oat groats and organic wheat for the bread if you think you may want to try making your own healthy bread.

Today, you can find organic canned beans and lentils in many grocery stores. *Eden* is a good organic canned brand. Always read the labels and make sure that the cans contain *only* what you expect. Never settle for soy in any form except in soy sauce where the soy is fermented and doesn't damage your family's health the way other soy products do. This means, other than soy sauce, *no soy* of *any kind* appears in *any food* you *ever buy.*

Soy is an estrogen enhancer. I don't want to sound silly, but at the same time soy disrupts hormones greatly so I want to issue more of a dire warning than I might otherwise do: You should feed your teenage boys soy products *only* if you want them to have the upper-body strength of their toddler sisters. I say this as a joke, but I'm also being serious. And the negative effects of soy on girls and women are just as bad in other ways. You have too many food choices to settle on risky soy. If you buy a can of beans, even organic, even *Eden*'s brand, read the labels because some contain soy fillers.

> **Note:** If you can add one more caution to your grocery chores, watch the plastic you use for food and drinks. Plastic can contain toxins known as *BPA.* Canned vegetables often come in plastic-lined cans, but many organic products are now offering canned beans and other organic vegetables in BPA-free cans. *Look for those and buy only those if you have the option.*

> **Note:** If there is any way to replace them, toss out all your aluminum cookware and Teflon-lined pans when you replace your plastic storage containers and water pitchers. Instead, do your best to cook with metal, cast iron, glass, and ceramic cookware and use similar kinds of storage containers. A good rule of thumb is this: If your great grandmother didn't cook on it or store food in it, you shouldn't either.

GABA likes the dopamine and serotonin standby foods too, such as the animal proteins and dairy so by including those foods for a healthy and lean body you're doing GABA a favor just as you are the others.

Wait a Minute! I Just Realized I Haven't Seen Fruit Listed Yet!

That's right you have not.

I love fruit. I also love Mounds and Almond Joy chocolate bars and corn on the cob and mashed potatoes. But I eat all of those sparingly. And for me, *sparingly* means – literally – maybe once every month or even less frequently.

For the most part, fruit does contain lots of good vitamins and minerals. That is the idea at least. The reality is that much of the fruit that gets to our tables were picked green, sprayed with pesticides, and rode in trucks for hundreds or thousands of miles ripening not on the vine but in an enclosed box.

This isn't your great grandmother's fruit.

For the most part, avoid all fruit juice. If you have a good blender such as a Vita-Mix and you make smoothies once in a while with *whole, organic fruit* and add greens to it like dark-green romaine lettuces, kale, the fiber in the resulting smoothie will help slow the absorption of bad sugar carbs in the fruit. And certainly whole, real fruit is a far better way to satisfy a sugar craving than any candy or ice cream.

Many fruits are especially beneficial to us such as berries and GABA likes mangoes and grapefruit and figs so they're certainly a viable option for your GABA needs. Acetylcholine also benefits from berries. Fruits that are multi-colored, especially berries, are fine even on a daily basis. Plus your brain and body will benefit from the anti-oxidant nature of berries.

But always treat most fruit like a special food. You don't have to avoid fruit as much as you avoid desserts and starchy vegetables, but you should *limit* your family's fruit intake.

In addition, if it's juice that you didn't squeeze, treat it like soy – just say no.

Acetylcholine and Food

Acetylcholine really enjoys complex carbs as well as fats that you get from nuts and seeds. B-vitamin foods improve acetylcholine levels. Yes, and no matter how much you've heard against a low-carb lifestyle or if you're not a meat eater (if not, have you ever wondered why your brain may be out of whack?) then you have to face facts and understand that the last brain chemical of the Fantastic Four, acetylcholine, benefits from your consumption of good, healthy grass-fed beef.

You can boost your body's production of acetylcholine levels through these kinds of foods:

- Beef
- Nuts, especially almonds and hazelnuts
- Berries and cherries
- Green, leafy vegetables
- Colorful vegetables
- Peanuts
- Fats from oils such as olive oil, fish oil, cod liver oil, coconut oil, and macadamia nut oil (yum!)
- Butter – Yep, grass-fed butter that you should now already have due to the 10-Hour Coffee Diet!
- Fish, including shrimp due to its high omega-3 content

It seems that the omega-3 oils in fish benefit acetylcholine in a greater way than the others. You can also get good quantities of omega-3 from flaxseed oil, but some flaxseed oil is said to produce an estrogen effect. Don't be afraid of flaxseed oil if you are male, but buy fresh, organic flaxseeds from stores such as Whole Foods and grind the seeds right before you eat them or put them over a salad or in a veggie green smoothie. The flaxseed that you grind and eat right away (or eat whole) is great.

Fiber-filled foods such as beans and lentils help to detox and clean out body's sewage system. This frees up your body's resources to work more effectively at creating brain chemicals and controlling your weight. You can add psyllium husks to your smoothies to help add some bulk if you need more fiber. Your body will tell you whether you need more fiber. The lentils and beans are not only a great source of fiber, but they add the benefit of bringing you a lot of protein also.

You should have at least 35 grams of fiber a day. The average American gets around 10 grams. If you're not having two or more bowel movements a day, then you're probably not getting enough fiber. If you already get a lot of fiber and still see a problem (or you have the opposite issue with diarrhea more than every once in a while) you might be getting too much fiber. If so, cut back on the psyllium if you've been adding it. Cut back on the fiber-heavy foods as a secondary step if you still need to do so.

12

YOUR BODY AND BRAIN'S INTERACTION WITH FOOD

Every time you eat or drink, you change your body's chemical make-up in some way.

Your Body and Brain on Fats

In addition to traditional food you can boost your brain's health through certain fats, spices, and liquids. We've covered some of the fats already (such as nuts and avocados and flaxseed), but it's worth looking at the effects these can have on your brain in more detail. Shortly, we'll look at spices and liquids as they are additional prongs in a multi-pronged approach to eating right, feeling better, and boosting your brain.

Keep in mind that not all fats are equal. The fat in a caramel-based, milk chocolate candy bar and the fat in cheap, store-bought beef can be bad for you for different reasons. The fat in the candy is fat from non-food and from partially hydrogenated trans fat sources can raise your LDL cholesterol (the "bad" cholesterol) and lower your HDL cholesterol (the "good" cholesterol) among other things. The fat in corn-fed beef that was fed hormones and antibiotics from cradle to grave contains the toxins injected into the cattle.

The Fats

The good fats, the ones you almost surely need more of include fat sources such as:

- Grass-fed, animal sources
- Olive oil (always buy olive oil in dark, glass containers and always get the extra virgin kind)
- Organic coconut oil (always buy organic, extra virgin coconut oil)

- Macadamia nut oil (these last three oils are wonderful to cook with, even eggs are great cooked in all of them although I cook my eggs in organic coconut oil)
- Egg yolks (*never* eat just the egg whites; complete eggs are one of the most perfect foods and you need yolks that are never overcooked; the better you source your eggs (such as from a local farmer – go to a local farmer's market -- who lets his chickens roam free daily) the better the eggs will be for your brain and body)
- Fish and fish oil supplements (we'll discuss supplements later)
- Fresh, ground flaxseed oil
- Organic nuts and seeds
- Grass-fed butter
- Avocados

Note: To be safe, avoid any and all products sold as being "fat free." Much of these products include hidden sugars (rarely does the label say "sugar" or we wouldn't be fooled into buying them).

The idea is always to decrease bad fats (best to eliminate them altogether) and increase your intake of the good fats.

A Word about Salad Dressing

You'll probably eat more salads as you improve your brain. The green leafy and other colored vegetables in salads are great. Salad dressings do contain fat unless you make the unhealthy mistake of ordering or buying "fat free" dressing. Still, most salad dressings these days contain so much sugar or soy and other horrid ingredients that you should avoid them unless you make your own or carefully scan a health food store's products to get the best kind you can find.

Consider this: take your own extra virgin olive oil, in its dark glass container, with you when you eat out and ask for your salads dry or dressing on the side. I was surprised that I enjoyed salads with only healthy olive oil and some added salt (I also have with me Celtic brand or Real Salt sea salt). If you do too, this is an extremely healthy way to eat salad and get needed, healthy fat.

I'll talk more about salt shortly.

Don't Go Nuts with the Nuts!

Nuts are sometimes called "domino foods" because we eat a "few" of them and a few minutes later we look down at an empty can that was full when we started! Over-consuming nuts is easy to do. When you eat nuts, go to your cabinet and grab a moderate portion and walk away. Consider that the nuts in your hand are the only nuts you'll eat before your next meal and stick to that. You'll therefore get plenty of nuts and add great fat to your brain without overdoing it so as to affect your waistline.

Note: Again, get those glass jars with rubber gasket seals to store your nuts in. Also, keep them out of the sun. Don't go overboard and buy too many nuts at one time because they go rancid quicker than you might guess. As long as you keep them in a dark place and stored in sealed, glass containers (stay away from BPA-laden plastic containers) you can buy a couple of months' worth of nuts at a time. Don't buy more than that or they will begin to go rancid before you finish and before you even notice.

Again, the more work you use to source nuts (organic if possible always!) the more effective they will work on your brain and body because your body won't be fighting the pesticides.

A variety is usually better than eating only one kind. My only strong advice when choosing nuts is to always include organic almonds and Brazil nuts. Both are wonderful for you. Brazil nuts are an excellent source of selenium, but if you eat more than five or six a day they can become toxic to your body. Don't let this scare you into not eating them! Selenium is great for you and causes the Brazil nut to be a "complete" protein and extremely healthy in doses of up to six a day. For most people, four Brazil nuts daily will give you an ample supply of selenium although your annual blood tests will let you know for sure if you're getting enough selenium.

> **Note:** If you find yourself waking up in the middle of the night and can't go back to sleep, you may very well not be getting enough fat before bedtime. Before brushing your teeth tonight, grab a few Brazil nuts or almonds and eat them.

Here's another reason to welcome more healthy fat into your diet. Fat slows down the effects of weight-encouraging foods. Whereas the carbs in bread and chips will make you hungrier before a meal, if you eat a few nuts or a little fresh-ground flaxseed before a meal, the response of any carbs in that meal will be reduced due to the reduction in the glycemic response of that food.

Your Body and Brain on Spices

It was probably Dr. Braverman, M.D., who made the largest impact on the brain-aware nutrition industry when it comes to using spices (and teas) for improving brain health and thereby balancing not just your brain, but also your entire body.

Many spices are great for your brain's health and your body's balance. They also do two things:

- They give food more taste
- They stack the advantages of an already healthy diet!

In other words, once you begin to eat well, if you then add spices to your food the health benefits will be multiplied by the spices. You will lose weight *faster,* for example, if you eat a healthy, low-carb diet *with* spices such as cayenne pepper and turmeric than if you do not include those spices.

Eating a half-teaspoon of red chili flakes before a meal decreases the average caloric intake by about 15%. That 15% adds up over time to a lot of calories that your body and mind don't have to deal with.

Spices and herbs maximize nutrient density. They create a more thermogenic diet that makes you younger and healthier due to their medicinal-like properties. Spices can increase your feeling of fullness so you'll eat less. They also help you to eliminate adding too much salt, High Fructose Corn Syrup-based ketchup, worthless ground cardboard called "pepper," and other awful condiments to your meals.

You Refuse to Eat Hot, Spicy Food?

What's that? You hate hot, spicy food? The nerve of some people!

Many who now love hot spices didn't always. A preference for hot, spicy food *can easily be acquired.* Start slowly and over time add more. Perhaps just a sprinkle of cayenne pepper in a soup would be a good way to start. In just a few weeks you will demand more "hotness" in your food because your thighs will look hotter, but also because you'll actually crave it. Your brain's chemicals will crave more because of all the good that hot spices do for your brain.

If there is just no way you're going to use any of the hot spices no matter how much I try to convince you... or if you're certain you have a health problem that will be affected negatively from hot spices such as cayenne pepper... that's okay. Don't add the hotter spices to your food. There are plenty of other good spices to enjoy without forcing yourself to eat the hotter ones.

> **Note:** I'm aware that stomach issues come into play. Heartburn might be a historical problem for you. But if those purple pills (*Prilosec* and equivalents), the heartburn tablets, could be considered a food group for you as much as you have to take them, consider this: When you begin eating a low-carb, high protein, high healthy fat, and yes, a high amount of hot spicy foods, it's likely that you will have less and less heartburn over time until it goes away for good. So you owe it to yourself to try new spices in spite of problems in the past. Once you begin to eat brain-healthy and body-healthy foods and you drop the carbs and raise the fat and protein for a few days, try some spices that you used to think gave you heartburn.

If you have no true health reasons not to try hot spices, even if you just don't think you can handle them, try them slowly over time. Remember, the more you can get used to and consume hot spices on your food the faster your metabolism will be and the more weight you'll lose and most important, the faster your brain chemicals will increase.

Heartburn Revisited

Speaking of heartburn… if you still suffer with it, even after you begin enjoying a healthy eating routine, don't reach for the pills right away. Try something else instead.

Get a bottle of *Bragg Apple Cider Vinegar* and pour a cap full into a glass of water. Hold your nose if you have to and drink it. Or just take a sip straight from the bottle. Although vinegar seems acidic, it will neutralize heartburn most of the time. A bit before a meal or right after will aid in your digestion.

Vinegar is a fermented food and Bragg's is extra special in that it contains the "mother," bits of the original source from which it was fermented in to help its enzymes work better than the cheap, Heinz and other generic vinegars you can find. Stack your body's health benefits from vinegar by tossing out the other stuff and stick with Bragg.

Note: Later, I dedicate an entire chapter in this book to Apple Cider Vinegar.

Spices for Your Brain

Spices are difficult to pin down for a specific benefit because they offer so many benefits for the brain and body. Almost every recommended spice provides an assortment of benefits. From increasing metabolism to helping lower blood pressure to making foods taste unique and exciting to boosting your brain's chemicals like never before, spices are one of the most under-utilized dietary tools we have today.

Buying Spices

And with online purchasing made so easy, you can get a tremendous array of healthy, organic spices at far cheaper prices than ever before. Plus, if you live in a small town or a long distance from a health food store or grocery such as Whole Foods, it makes a lot of sense to order your spices online. You'll save money and gasoline and time by searching for them online.

> **Note:** I'd guard against ordering spices in the hotter, summer months. Even two- or three-day shipments means that your spices can sit in a hot postal facility for many hours at a time and run in a hot delivery truck far longer than they should. Even if your area is having a cool summer, other areas of the country might not be and you shouldn't risk ordering then. Plus, if a spice seller lives in the next state and both your state and that one are having a cool summer, did you know that – at least this was true in the past – *every single* FedEx package goes through the Tennessee FedEx hub before being delivered no matter where the sender and receiver live? This enables FedEx to ship as efficiently and cheaply as possible and I'm all for that, but keep this in mind when ordering food or spices online because you don't want a hot Tennessee summer to damage anything. So plan ahead and order your spices in the spring, fall, or winter, to ensure they arrive as fresh and potent as possible.

I'd like to section out the spices and tell you which brain chemicals they work best on, but they all seem to do some good in many ways so I'll just give you a list of spices that you should immediately add to your food pantry. With each spice I'll mention some extras about it to give you an idea of use or to describe one of its benefits that you might not have ever known or thought about.

It's been said that spices are "nutrient dense." Each one can provide 25 to 75 different nutrients for your brain and body.

The best advice I can give you initially, though, is to look in your spice rack and throw away everything more than a year old. Just toss it. It'll seem to hurt your wallet at first, but many spices go bad, stale, or at best inert even if they still taste okay after a year and sometimes even sooner. You want to stack every health advantage you can, right? So replace them.

Use the following general rules of thumb when getting spices:

- If you can grow the spice, it's always better than buying it no matter how fresh you can buy it. Spices aren't watermelons and you don't need lots of room for a spice garden. You can grow some spices indoors, you can have a small dirt box on a window sill and grow a few there, or just a 3x3 foot tilled soil using only organic fertilizer will produce far more than most families will ever consume through the growing season.
- If you grow your own, learn how to dry them so you and your family will have healthy spices year-round.
- If you buy them, always get organic if money isn't an issue. Don't skimp on your health to save a few dollars. When it comes to health you either pay now or you pay later. It's cheaper, and better for your health, to pay now than paying for it later with health problems and medical costs.
- Date your spices. When you buy a spice, write the date on the label. In a year, if you haven't eaten all that spice, toss it and buy its replacement.
- Buying a whole spice that you grate, such as garlic cloves and ginger root and cinnamon sticks is always better than buying pre-ground spices.
- When buying spices, don't buy them in the summer for the reasons listed earlier. Consider this: Don't even buy them at a health food store or Whole Foods-like grocery store in the summer! Your store will have had them delivered by truck or parcel so your store's supply faces the same summer heat conditions you face if you order them from home. Buying in spring is best because the previous summer-shipped stock sold out long ago and the stock on the shelves never saw hot months.
- Store your spices in a cool, dark cabinet.

The Array of Spices You Need Right Now

You may have noticed already, I often like to use bulleted lists because it helps you and I pinpoint specifics. I'm going to do the same when discussing individual spices next. I'll list each spice and then give you a summary of its benefits:

- Turmeric: Helps add smooth pathways to your brain's connections by reducing brain plaque. This boosts your avoidance of increased memory problems that can result in Alzheimer's disease. I love turmeric on eggs and meat of any kind.
- Cinnamon: An all-time favorite! As with Brazil nuts, cinnamon will add tremendous benefits to your health, but you *can* overdose on it so keep your consumption to no more than about 2 teaspoons daily. (This is an ample supply that allows you to use a lot throughout the day while still being in the safe zone.) Cinnamon is wonderful in coffee and tea *and it is fine to put cinnamon in your 10-Hour Coffee Diet Coffee!* Cinnamon also will *slow harmful effects of sugar in your blood stream.* If you are at a special moment where you are having a rare, sweet treat such as ice cream or pie, sprinkle cinnamon all over the dish and then enjoy your rare treat! Plus, cinnamon tastes good not only with sweet things, coffee, and tea, but also on other things including meat and chicken believe it or not. (Some love it on non-sweet things, some don't, but cinnamon's advantages are so incredible that it's worth learning all the foods you like cinnamon on to get more of it daily.) As with turmeric, cinnamon also helps our memory. If you can locate organic Saigon cinnamon and grind it yourself before you use it, you will maximize the effects of your cinnamon use more than any other way. Cinnamon tastes especially good on Greek and homemade yogurt.
- Basil: Basil is another spice that is simple to grow and provides a plethora of brain chemicals that improve dopamine.
- Black pepper: Not the stuff on the restaurant tables or store shelves. As long as you get real black pepper that you must grind you'll increase your metabolism and help your dopamine levels, but in addition, pepper greatly improves the effects of turmeric so why not stack your turmeric's benefits while you're at it?

- Garlic: Great for your heart, amazing for your immune system and wonderful for your brain chemicals! I am sad to announce that I have a problem with fresh garlic in that it breaks out a small bit of rosacea I sometimes get on my cheeks. So I have to get garlic in capsule form to give my brain as much as I want to give it. If you get garlic from capsules, be sure to get "odor-free" garlic capsules or your breath will smell as bad after the capsules as if you ate the raw cloves! Trust me on this.
- Sage: Another memory spice, perhaps the best available. Your brain will soak it up like a sponge.
- Cumin: Increases alertness and memory and tastes good too!
- Cilantro/Coriander: Helps detoxify your body and that frees up your body's resources to repair any damage and stay healthy and fight weight gain.
- Cayenne Pepper: Wonderful for metabolism, all four brain chemicals seem to prosper with it, and you'll feel better afterwards too. If you just can't take the pepper, you can get cayenne pepper in capsule form. By the way, spicy foods can ward off anxiety by calming your brain by boosting the Fantastic Four brain chemicals so it's definitely worth the effort to try the hotter spices and see how well you can get used to them. Cayenne pepper is one of my all-time favorite weight-loss enhancers and brain energizers. Did you know that cayenne pepper will even seal a serious open wound long enough, in many cases, to get a victim to the hospital that otherwise wouldn't make it? There is so much about hot cayenne that is cool that I am going to offer a sidebar section just on this spice alone before the chapter ends.
- Peppermint: Tastes great in so many teas and boosts your thought power as well as having somewhat of a boost to metabolism. Adding crushed peppermint leaves to your tea is far more effective in allowing your brain and body to utilize the spice than settling for "peppermint tea." Peppermint in a tea you drink following a meal helps you feel more satisfied and helps to ward off false "I'm still hungry" triggers that we sometimes get before our stomachs have had time to tell our brains that we actually are full.
- Ginger: Ginger tastes so good! And it reduces motion sickness, nausea, and even inflammation such as arthritis and back pain. Your brain loves it and your body does better with it. (Reduce your ginger intake if you're pregnant, as it has been shown to promote early contractions in some women.)
- Saffron: Boosts your mood by feeding your brain's serotonin. If you feel depressed, saffron will provide a pick-me-up.

Note: In addition to adding cinnamon to reduce the effects of bad carbs, eating bad carbs slowly causes them to affect you less negatively than wolfing them down. Savor the flavor of your cinnamon-sprinkled treat, take the time to taste each small bite, smell the aroma, and feel the texture on your tongue. Not only will you appreciate that treat far more, did you know that you would feel full much faster and not crave an immediate doubling-down of the same dish as we sometimes do? *And* the effects on our hips and thighs are greatly reduced when we eat bad carbs slowly.

If it's a common spice and not on the list above, add it to your food if you like it! I didn't provide an exhaustive list above. Nutmeg, spearmint, dill, allspice, anise, fennel, and so many more boost your brain and your body.

Combine spices all you want! All of these and other everyday, common spices are food and not drugs. I find that if I eat any food with onions, I can add cinnamon, garlic, ginger, and turmeric to ramp up the good "burn" I feel after that meal. Such a workhorse of revving-up spices seems to boost my energy and metabolism like no other.

While you might not want to carry a purse full of spices with you to every restaurant you eat at (especially if you're a guy), to the extent that you do that, you will be eating healthier, boosting the weight loss capability of a low-carb, high-protein diet, making your food taste better and more unique, and your brain will be swimming in wonderful dopamine, serotonin, GABA, and acetylcholine like never before.

Revisiting Cayenne Pepper

Earlier in this chapter I told you some of the great aspects of cayenne pepper. All of these spices are amazing and in the USA spices are severely underutilized. If the government wanted us all to improve our health, it would stop trying to take over the vitamin industry and provide public service announcements promoting the benefits of spices.

And the one that should get the most attention in my opinion is cayenne pepper.

I'm not the only one who holds that opinion. Recently, Dr. Al Sears, M.D., sent his email subscribers this note about this amazing life-boosting spice:

> *Most people think that hot spicy food is bad for your health. Yet in some cases, the exact opposite is true. Cayenne peppers can make your eyes water and your tongue burn, but they also have healing power.*
>
> *Several widely separated cultures have used cayenne for medicinal purposes for centuries. Now modern scientific research validates much of the folklore. Cayenne peppers can ward off the common cold and flu. They take away arthritic pain and help asthma sufferers. Cayenne pepper can stop itching and both internal and external bleeding. Cayenne peppers can help your body fend off ailments such as heart disease, cancers, cataracts, Alzheimer's disease and others.*
>
> *Today I'll show you how to use the naturally occurring, medicinal properties in cayenne peppers to improve your health.*
>
> *Cayenne contains a compound called capsaicin. Capsaicin is the ingredient that gives peppers their heat. Generally, the hotter the pepper, the more capsaicin it contains. In addition to adding heat to the pepper, capsaicin acts to reduce platelet stickiness and relieve pain. Research shows cayenne can help to:*

Improve Circulation. Cayenne peppers are a circulatory stimulant that facilitates blood flow. Used as a heart attack preventative, cayenne can do wonders in toning your heart and keeping it in top condition. Also, cayenne is one of the richest and most stable sources of Vitamin E, which is also cardio-protective.

Benefit Your Heart. Cayenne and other red chili peppers reduce triglyceride levels, and platelet aggregation, while increasing the body's ability to dissolve fibrin, a substance integral to the formation of blood clots. Cultures that liberally use hot peppers, like cayenne, have a much lower rate of heart attack, stroke and pulmonary embolism.

Fight Inflammation. Capsaicin is a potent inhibitor of substance P, a neuropeptide associated with inflammatory processes. When animals injected with a substance that causes arthritis ate capsaicin, they had significantly reduced inflammation. Other research shows that peppers can help control pain associated with arthritis, psoriasis, and diabetic neuropathy.

Clear Congestion. The peppery heat in capsaicin also stimulates secretions that help clear mucus from your stuffed up nose or congested lungs. Capsaicin is similar to a compound found in many cold remedies for breaking up congestion, except that capsaicin works much faster. A tea made with hot cayenne pepper very quickly stimulates the mucus membranes lining the nasal passages to drain, helping to relieve congestion and stuffiness.

Boost Immunity. Cayenne also helps maintain healthy epithelial tissues including the mucous membranes that line the nasal passages, lungs, intestinal tract and urinary tract and serve as the body's first line of defense against invading pathogens.

Prevent Stomach Ulcers. Cayenne peppers have a bad – and undeserved – reputation for contributing to stomach ulcers. Not only do they ***not*** cause ulcers, these hot peppers may help prevent them by killing harmful bacteria and stimulating the stomach to secrete protective buffering juices that prevent ulcer formation. The use of cayenne pepper is actually associated with a reduced risk of stomach ulcers. It stimulates peristalsis and emptying of the stomach.

Drop A Few Extra. That heat you feel after eating hot peppers takes energy and calories to produce. Cayenne peppers contain substances called capsinoids that significantly increase thermogenesis (heat production) and oxygen consumption in your fat tissue after you eat them.

If you like to eat peppers, don't listen to the "naysayers." Hot Mexican, Szechwan, Indian, or those smoldering Thai dishes can make excellent choices.

You'll be amazed at how easy it is to incorporate cayenne into your cuisine. I tend to use cayenne by taste and add it to my food in place of black pepper. It is also quite good in salsa.

I also keep a bottle of cayenne in my house for emergencies. The other day, I was cutting down some bananas and accidentally cut my hand with a machete. I sprinkled some cayenne on the cut, applied pressure and the bleeding stopped immediately.

You can also get cayenne in supplement form. Try to get a capsule of at least 500mg, with at least 40,000 heat units, although some may have up to 100,000 heat units.[55]

Your Body and Brain on Liquids

Any discussion of brain/body performance would be incomplete without talking about liquids. Liquids are a part of our diet, but we tend to forget that aspect. We tend to ignore the liquids we consume when we focus on what is good for us.

I want to help you seal in your mind that your daily diet includes the food, the spices, and the liquids you consume. Liquids affect everything just as the spices and food do. Your body is a system of parts that work together to produce results. Your brain and body need fat and liquid for proper lubrication and waste elimination.

Healthy Fruit Juices and Diet Sodas Are Neither!

We've already covered the dangerous infusion of fructose sugar that drives into your system when you drink fruit juice. This is especially true for fruit juice that you don't make in a blender where you keep all the fruit's fiber that helps slow down the fruit sugar.

Stay away from fruit juice.

In general, treat fruit juices like special dessert treats. If you make green smoothies with some fruit and green veggies, go heavier on the greens and use berries for most of the fruit.

Diet sodas contain heavy amounts of aspartame. Have you noticed what kind of soda most overweight people seem to drink? It's almost always diet soda! Some may say that is because they're overweight and they're trying to reduce calories so you can't blame diet sodas when in fact they may have mistakenly turned to diet sodas thinking they'll help lose weight. Maybe. But diet sodas encourage hunger pangs. The acid destroys good flora in your gut. Your brain gets nothing from it, but still has to process the unnatural chemicals you put into your body every time you drink a can or (ugh!) a 2-liter bottle of the stuff. If you were overweight before starting on diet sodas, you can be assured that diet sodas won't do anything to get you to lose weight and usually do the exact opposite and cause you to gain even more weight.

Water, Water Everywhere and Not a Drop to Drink

I already sound like an extreme nut probably so I won't go into my usual diatribe about the water we drink, but let me just offer a few nuggets of advice or I won't feel as though I've done you right.

Municipal water is bad. Maybe I will go into my diatribe.

Municipal water being bad means the water that comes out of that tap in your kitchen is bad. The water that comes out of your shower faucet is bad. Municipal water contains chlorine and fluoride and lots of other things (as if chlorine and fluoride weren't bad enough) that slowly ebb away your body's ability to fight immunities and other problems.

What About Cavities?

Any water department official, upon hearing that fluoride is bad for our health, and any traditional, ADA-approved dentist is going to go crazy if you ever bad-mouth fluoride. They immediately tell you how cavities are reduced in a fluoride-rich environment.

That is true.

Cavities result from a growth of bacteria in your mouth that occurs in everybody to some extent. If you don't regularly clean your mouth and teeth, the bacteria can grow and cause a rotting of your teeth. Yech!

Not to change the subject (because I am not) but do you know what a major ingredient of rat poison is? Good old fluoride! Fluoride kills rats and mice. Fluoride *does* help kill bacteria in your mouth, but so would battery acid. So will ammonia. So will bleach. Want to brush your teeth with Clorox bleach? Why not, it'll kill bacteria that cause cavities.

Note: Not wanting to rinse with Clorox is also a reason not to want chlorine in your family's drinking water. Chlorine is a harsh chemical that your body fights and cannot use to its benefit. Also note that your skin, your body's biggest organ, soaks up chlorine when you go swimming in chlorinated pools.

Do you know why even the dental profession warns parents against using fluoride toothpaste in toddlers' mouths? It's because toddlers will swallow some of the toothpaste. That can kill a baby just as it kills a big rat. How do you like this continued reference to rats, poison, and babies? I don't like the connection either. That is why I warn you strongly against allowing fluoride anywhere close to you or your family's mouths.

Burt's Bees, *Dr. Collins*, and *Tom's* are makers of fluoride-free toothpastes and you can find other brands in health food stores and online. Even better, mix up some baking soda and hydrogen peroxide and use that when you brush. Whatever you do, stop *today* using fluoride-based products like toothpastes and mouth rinses. And stop using the fluoridated water too

Filtration

Not drinking tap water produces some challenges. It means that all your cooking, all your tea and coffee, and anything else you make with water that goes into your body has to be from a non-municipal source.

What you can do is get a filtration system. If you get a reverse osmosis whole house system (Google it) you'll make *all* your water healthier, chlorine and fluoride-free, and even your showers will be healthy finally. As Dr. Joseph Mercola, M.D. warns, in many ways municipal water that comes out of the shower is *worse for us* than the same water we drink. Our skin is the largest organ of our bodies and the skin absorbs the water's chemicals as it passes over our bodies during a shower. Unfortunately, the chemicals we absorb in the shower don't expel through urination.

Whether it's worse to shower or drink it is not something I care about either way. I don't want any of it.

You shouldn't either.

Until you get a whole house system? Get a filter that does the same thing. Some of the Brita filter systems are nice and come in pitchers that filter water. Make sure you get them molded in BPA-free plastic. My all-time favorite larger, stand-alone, non-electric water filter is the Berkey filter (Berkeyfilters.com). You get a stainless-steel *or* BPA-free plastic Berkey system with heavy-duty ceramic filters that rarely need changing.

You can put red food coloring in water, run it through the Berkey, and it comes out crystal clear!

Drink water throughout your day, every day, and drink pure, clean water instead of the stuff you get from the faucet. If your brain needs lots and lots of water to be healthy, and if your body needs lots and lots of water to be healthy, why on earth are you doing hesitating on this?

Drinking Out

A lot of restaurants actually filter their water to some degree. Often, the icemakers use water filters and the drinking water they serve is filtered. But certainly the water isn't filtered to get rid of all the chlorine and fluoride… it's because of taste reasons. The taste of municipal water doesn't always blend well with soda syrups and teas and coffees.

Still, you're better off not drinking water or tea when you eat out. But yes, I do and my family does. At least the coffee and tea has been brewed somewhat. If you don't want to bring your own drink, and some places won't even let you if you wanted to, here's a tip: just let a glass of ice water sit on your table for a while before you reach for it. Some of the chlorine actually leaves the water into the air.

Amazingly, they make a drinking water filter *straw* (amazon.com/Seychelle-Water-Filter-Straw-

Advanced/dp/accessories/B003U4PQ84) that you can use to filter water when you eat out. This doesn't do you much good if you order tea or coffee, but it's certainly better than not using it and drinking the water directly.

Note: Keep in mind that vegetables and berries are mostly water. As you move away from a fast-food eating regimen and towards a low-carb, high protein, high fat, leafy and colorful vegetable diet you naturally consume more liquids in your foods, especially the produce. Still, you should make it a point to drink fresh, clean water every time you think of it. People used to bash the Atkins Diet for being bad on your kidneys given its heavy protein advice. I recall that Gary Taubes in the book *Good Calories, Bad Calories* (a good book loaded with extremely advanced scientific studies) shows that the protein kidney scare is just that, a scare, but with a lot of protein you do need to drink more fluids to stay lubricated and well hydrated as opposed to a high-carb diet that includes are more sugary fruits.

A Good Water Strategy to Ward Off Overeating

If you are on the off day of your 10-Hour Coffee Diet or feeling extremely hungry and temped to splurge on something bad, drink water 30 minutes before your meal and you should feel more full and eat less. When your urine color is light yellow to clear, it means you're getting enough water. Water from food counts towards your overall water intake. If you take a lot of vitamin supplements your urine will be darker and more yellow because you can't help but eliminate some excess supplements after you take them. Your body rarely absorbs all of a vitamin whether that vitamin comes from food or from a supplement.

Note: Your urine may be darker the first time you urinate each day due to not drinking water while you slept. That's fine. Judge whether you're getting enough water from your urine color starting with the second time you urinate each day and throughout the day after that.

Tea and Coffee

The caffeine in coffee and tea can stimulate your brain's chemicals. That's the case with the 10-Hour Coffee Diet coffee (or tea). The bottom line seems to be that just about any tea will boost your brain's chemicals and stimulate your metabolism so a glass with your dinner sounds like a delight.

When to Drink Tea for Maximum Effects

Nutrients in teas are said to speed up your metabolism. Green tea can reduce absorption of bad fats you eat by as much as 40%. The best time actually to maximize your tea's effectiveness is to drink it after a meal. (Even drinking tea right after a fast food meal is going to help your body handle that bad fat.)

Some research shows that Yerba Mate and Oolong tea are great for their effects on metabolism and fat limitation. In addition, Rooibos tea has far more antioxidants then the typical green tea.

13

PHYSICAL MANIFESTATIONS OF HEALTHY AND NUTRIENT-DEPRIVED BRAINS

So many topics seem to come out of brain nutrition.

Tackle Your Cravings for Salty Foods

Sometimes we just *need* salted, buttered popcorn. Right?

Salt Cravings

Serotonin deficiency leads to salt cravings. Fix your brain... fix your body.

Without excess salt intake, you won't get bloated or excess water retention. You'll lose water weight immediately. Having too many salty foods creates a craving for even more salty foods. Eliminate or drastically reduce salty foods and your cravings for them go away.

Use spices to make this happen. If you want salt on your food because of taste, the spices mentioned earlier can dramatically reduce or eliminate your desire for salt.

Still, Stop Slamming Salt!

In spite of all I just told you, I'm not down on salt *in general.*

Some heart patients need to reduce salt. But salt is not bad for your heart in general and for a healthy society we need to look at some truth behind this condiment that is a required part of a healthy diet.

Like red meat, fat, and the sun, salt has gotten a bad rap. Your brain and body need an ample supply of sodium to function properly. When you begin to eat better you will eat fewer candy bars and fast foods because your brain will want fewer of those kinds of things. Your sodium intake will go from a high amount of bad, processed, white salt to not enough salt.

Get salt and use it! Don't be afraid of it, especially as you eat higher quality foods that won't have as much sodium as the foods you used to binge on. As I mentioned earlier, I carry with me either Celtic brand or Real Salt brand. Of the two, my preference is the Real Salt brand. I get it on Amazon.com.

I only let my family eat "sea salt." Sea salt is unprocessed (if you buy a good brand) and doesn't look uniformly white and is not as uniformly ground as the white, processed salt. That is good and you should expect it. You will also find that it tastes much better than the typical salt. It's also much healthier for your brain and body than traditional table salt.

Tackle Your Cravings for Sweet Foods

In my opinion, a far more dangerous craving than salt is a sugar. Spices don't fulfill sugar cravings as easily as they fulfill salt cravings due to their more tangy taste.

We desire sweets because we like them. Eating sweets can be a good thing. Berries and tropical fruits are good for us. The problem is that we tend to overeat sweets like crazy. And if only the sweets that we did overeat were limited strictly to fruits, we'd still have some problems, but far fewer than we do today with obesity, diabetes, heart disease, and slower brain connections.

Sweets Drive Sweets

The more carbohydrates we eat, especially simple carbohydrates, the more we desire. This is one reason why a low-carb diet will decrease your desire for sweets.

When it comes to the brain, it is serotonin that is released whenever we eat carbohydrates. Most of us *really* like candy bars and ice cream because of the immediate rush that we get which is nothing more than a release of serotonin in our brains that makes us feel good. Remember, serotonin is the Happy chemical.

We have all been rewarded with sweets as children growing up. Each birthday is a happy occasion associated with wonderful ice cream and cake. Often, when we get a promotion at work or something special happens, someone will throw us a little party and have a cake or some sort of dessert. Children are rewarded with cookies when they do something special. In today's affluent world, so are our dogs!

> **Note:** We do our pets no more justice than we do our children by feeding them sugar-laden treats, thinly disguised as "dog treats" on the packages.

Avoiding Sweets

Again, one of the best ways to avoid sugar cravings is to start and stay with a high-fat, protein-rich, low-carb eating plan. Consider this a lifelong plan, not a temporary diet. (Just to be clear, the 10-Hour Coffee Diet is a plan you can use for the rest of your life.) In doing so, your four brain chemicals will automatically boost up, which makes your serotonin higher. This makes you happier and more fulfilled, and that eliminates one place that sugar has been used in your life: that is, you will not feel the need to have sugar as a reward for something because you already feel rewarded through your everyday diet.

> **Note:** There is a psychological advantage to going all out if you *do* decide to eat a dessert. When you finally give in to a sweet craving, really give in to it! Go all out, and buy a high-quality item. (Never keep desserts at home to avoid temptation.) So when you do finally reward yourself with a dessert, it is a decadent, high-quality dessert that you can savor and eat slowly and really enjoy.

Exercise

I will talk later about the connection between exercise, your brain, and your body, but sometimes I actually get up and walk around the house, or go outside and walk around my home a couple of times, and my craving for sugar actually goes away completely.

Why is that?

You should be able to guess at the answer already. Even though we haven't discussed exercise yet, you probably suspect by now that exercise boosts your brain chemicals. All of the Fantastic Four brain chemicals are helped by exercise, even a small amount of exercise. When you feel satisfaction in your mind, your body feels good to, and you lose the sugar reward desire that you might have had before.

Medications – Poisons or Prizes?

There is very little I plan to say here. I've said most of it before now.

Most everybody reading this book can fix their brain and their body almost always, except in cases where things have progressed too far or due to rare genetics, by food and supplementation.

The Real Crime – Supplements Considered Drugs

Soon it may get to the point where the lobbyists for drug manufacturers will get the government to regulate the supplement industry. You see; the drug manufacturers don't like competition... and they have a powerful lobby in Washington, D.C. If the supplement industry ever does get regulated, it may mean you won't be able to buy natural supplements without prescriptions. Instead of allowing freedom of choice for people, the government would basically regulate natural supplements out of business to the benefit of the pharmaceutical industry.

The FDA

I discussed earlier about how bad of a job the FDA/USDA does in teaching Americans about the proper way to eat and about good nutrition. The famous food pyramid needs to be turned upside down because it is exactly, 100%, the opposite advice that you should be getting for a healthy mind and body.

The government is smart. Recently, the government decided to replace the food pyramid with a different design using a colorful, segmented plate with food on it. They realized many people are warning against the food pyramid. So what did they do? They changed the food pyramid into something that's not a pyramid. It's a food plate. The results are just as disastrous as the food pyramid that we've had for decades: "Grains are your friends, meat is your enemy."

It didn't really get better.

Side Effects of Drugs

The average drug today has 70 official side effects.

Have you ever watched TV and saw a commercial about a drug and it lists all the side effects for that drug. About an hour later, a commercial for a different drug appears that fixes the side effects from the drug shown earlier!

Dr. Joel Robbins, a homeopathic doctor in Tulsa, Oklahoma has said the following for years (paraphrased for brevity):

> *"If you take a drug but you are not sick, you will get sick. A drug is a poison. The poison is designed to specifically attack one thing without regard for any other damage it might do."*

If you haven't seen 70 side effects on the sides of drugs you've taken recently, that's because there simply is not room. On average, Dr. William Campbell Douglass, M.D., states that there are actually *five times* more side effects than what is on the typical label of any drug for sale today.

The side effects pile up, sometimes exponentially, when you take more than one.

So... you're low on serotonin. You can quickly fix it little by little through food and dietary supplements such as sprinkling saffron spice on your chicken.

Or you can take oxytocin and antidepressants, drugs that increase serotonin. The FDA says that, other than 70 or so side effects of each of those drugs, you might be helped.

If you can get off the stuff when you're done!

There are *not* 70 known side effects for saffron.

There are *not* 70 known side effects for B-12, a good supplement for serotonin deficiency.

There are *not* 70 known side effects for turkey, a food that boosts serotonin levels through the roof.

So, *why* would anyone consider a drug for serotonin? Promise me you won't be someone who does.

Consider Chelation

Toxins in your system, especially heavy metals, work against your body. Some can last until you reach the grave (and depending on the amount of toxins, that can be sooner than later I'm sad to say). Your body constantly works to get around and to fight those toxins and the more your body does that, the fewer resources are available for beneficial processes such as producing dopamine, serotonin, GABA, and acetylcholine.

If you feel chronically blah, and you're eating well and using good teas and spices, consider finding a local doctor who performs chelation therapy and get tested for heavy metals. You might have toxins that your body cannot get rid of. Mercury from amalgam fillings and vaccines can stay in your cells and do their damage slowly over time if you don't get rid of it.

If you test and learn you have heavy metals, often a doctor can rid you of them in a few chelation sessions. They sound far worse than they are. I've had them. You get an IV for an hour and a half about 6 times. The IV contains vitamins and also binding agents for the toxins such as mercury and lead that might be in your system. You will eliminate those toxins when you urinate because of their binding to the IV vitamins and supplements such as MSM that you'll take during the time you receive the chelation.

A final test will show you are free from the toxins, or perhaps you might need a few more chelation sessions. Either way, you will soon enough be rid of toxins that come in the insidious form of heavy metals, perhaps for the first time in your adult life. Your brain and body will be dramatically freed up because your cells will be communicating nicely for the first time in a long while.

If you're sick or feel down more than you should, you either need to:

- Feed yourself something you're lacking or
- Get rid of something you have too much of.

If the food and supplements in this book don't boost your brain and body, get tested right away for toxins in the form of heavy metals.

> **Note:** You may very well have a serious disease that food, supplements, and chelation cannot solve. This is always possible, but for most people reading this book that simply isn't the case. That is, unless you go too long with those toxins in your body where their damage begins to be so severe it becomes permanent.

Don't reach for a prescription first. Make that your last resort.

Supplements Boost Your Brain Dramatically

Supplements have been the topic I've been most excited to tell you about.

Most books about the brain and body connection mention supplements but they don't do them justice. Supplements are often treated as an after-thought at best and as sort of an equal to drugs at worse.

If we could get all our needed vitamins and minerals from our food, I'd be against supplements. But the truth is that we cannot get our vitamins and minerals from the foods we eat in most cases. I will say that if you live on a farm, grow only high brix produce (see International Ag Labs), if you raise your own grass-fed cattle, raise free-range chickens, and create a recycle system where your animal waste becomes fertilizer and so on, then I would have to say: you probably don't need to supplement.

But this is not the year 1712. Most of us don't have the means to do all that.

We need to supplement because our food sources, no matter how much we attempt to make them good ones, cannot be as beneficial as we'd like them to be. I still strongly urge you to follow all of the advice we've given so far. But to balance your brain quickly, to get your body into the best shape possible, and to see results and *keep results*, you should also supplement the food you eat to maximize the Fantastic Four brain chemicals: dopamine, serotonin, GABA, and acetylcholine.

Supplements Provide Between-Meal Nutrients

After you eat, your body needs to digest your food. The reason most people eat every three or four hours is not because they get work breaks then. That time interval is needed, in general, to process and digest the previous meal, utilize the energy from it, store any excess in our fat stores, and prepare the stomach enzymes for the next wave of incoming food.

Before or between meals your body is doing its best to grab all the nutrients possible from the food you ate at your last meal. But you can use that downtime to boost the vitamins and minerals in your body and to energize more production of the Fantastic Four brain chemicals by supplementing your body.

There's another reason why you take supplements between or before meals. For most brain supplements, you should take them when food isn't fresh in your system because the supplements will get absorbed more quickly. Food can act as a blocking agent and make supplements far less effective. Given their expense you always want to stack as many advantages on top of other advantages as you can when supplementing so watch your timing.

The only brain supplements you'll want to take with food are ones with fat in them such as cod liver oil, fish oil, and or lecithin granules.

Not All Supplements Are Equal

You do often get what you pay for. Yes, you can go to Wal-Mart and get some of the supplements I recommend. Perhaps all of them are there. But many are made in China and the companies that farm out the work there do not perform nearly enough quality control to ensure the supplements are pure or even as safe as they should be.

Stack the advantages! I keep saying it because in life if you begin to see the arithmetic advantages to stacking whatever you do to squeeze additional benefits, you will soon learn that you are getting more results with less effort than ever before. And life's too short not to maximize our efforts, isn't it?

Lots of deals abound if you look. But I'm going to give you links to online sources where I get *my* supplements and tell you where and why. So I don't hesitate to tell you that and suggest that you do the same.

If you've been getting supplements elsewhere and you want to continue, more power to you. Unfortunately, I can only give these recommendations to people who live in the USA. If you live outside the USA, the shipping cost may be too prohibitive for you to get them. You will need to look online and in your local health food stores for similar supplements if you're not in the USA or can't buy these supplements from the USA and have them shipped to where you live.

Before Getting Specific

Supplements are not magic bullets. They sometimes seem to work wonders though.

Supplements will not necessarily be directly responsible for any of your weight loss even though they can help indirectly in so many ways. In addition, they provide nutrients that boost your brain's chemicals and your *brain* is mostly responsible for your weight loss. Keep in mind that is the fundamental principle of this entire book.

If you go to a traditional, cut-and-drug doctor, including most M.D.'s and D.O.'s, they might warn you against any supplementation. The common catchphrase they are taught early to say is often, "You'll just pee them all out... it is simpler to throw your money in the toilet." And of course they often follow that up with, "I can prescribe some safe drugs that might help" (while they pray you won't read the side effects on the packaging).

Still, I'd like to see you go to a doctor that is open to non-drug solutions instead of drug-gambling. If you find a doctor that performs chelation or one that offers an array of supplements on display when you walk into the waiting room, that doctor probably understands the risks of drugs and the hope of supplements. Seek this kind of doctor out.

I would strongly urge that you see a homeopath or naturalist, but I don't want to toss the baby out with the bathwater because a medical doctor can order blood tests and perform certain routines that the others might not always be able to do. So try to locate an M.D. or D.O. that shows a pro-active willingness to try alternative therapies and pass along your supplement list to see what he or she says about how your body might react and be helped by your supplement list. It's not only best, it's imperative to make sure that you don't have a hidden condition that would hamper or even counteract adversely with a supplement. It's difficult to stress how rare that would be versus an adverse reaction to just about any common drug prescribed tens of thousands of times daily, but you owe it to yourself and your family to dot your *i*'s and cross your *t*'s before starting your supplement regimen.

Supplements are a major start to the process of weight loss. Supplements "prime the pump" for weight loss. If diet and exercise are not working, it's possible that your brain may be blocking all your other weight loss efforts. These supplements help enhance and amplify your diet and exercise efforts for weight loss. They "unlock" your brain, freeing it up to handle your body better to flip the weight loss switch. But to be clear, these are NOT weight loss supplements.

Prime Your Brain's Weight Loss Program!

I tried several approaches to this chapter. I thought about breaking it into sections on dopamine, serotonin, GABA, and acetylcholine then list the supplements that boosted each one of those. The problem with that, as with spices, is that many of the supplements work across the spectrum on multiple brain chemicals but even more important, you need to approach supplements more from a holistic view.

You don't necessarily take a supplement to boost a specific brain chemical unless you know you're *severely* lacking in that one. Instead, boost all of them. These supplements work well together, some work extremely well in certain combinations. To shortcut your work and research, I'm going to reveal the punch line early! Like a *Columbo* episode that tells who the murderer is in the first few minutes instead of waiting for the end of the show, I'm going to describe two of the most amazing supplement combos that boost your brain in incredible ways.

I have a supplement combo that I have honed to almost pure perfection that I take in the morning and another that I take at night. It in no way requires any change to any of the 10-Hour Coffee Diet's protocols.

This supplement combo provides a tremendous performance enhancing, brain-boosting, chemical-jumpstart naturally without drugs. The supplements work with the fats and coffee and the meal I eat to give me a synergistic effect where the combination is more powerful than the sum of the parts.

I want things to be easy and simple for you. I get so frustrated at the books on diet, weight loss, exercise, and the brain when they put supplements all over the books and discuss *possible* combinations here and there. You have to keep going back, looking at the index and table of contents, just to get an initial shopping list of supplements and then you still aren't sure what and when you take them.

Not here. I want to give you answers. To boost your brain's chemical nutrients and maximize your weight loss and body tone, you'll take two specific supplement combinations.

Ready? Hang on as best you can.

The Morning Brainiac's Energizing Cocktail

Here is the recipe you need for the Morning Brainiac's Energizing Cocktail:

- Three grams of L-Tyrosine
- 300-600 mg of St. John's Wort
- One to two grams of L-Phenylalanine
- 100-200 mg of DMAE
- One and a half grams of Acetyl Carnitine

- One tablespoon of Lecithin granules
- 500 mcg of B-12

(I'll cover sources for these and describe each one in just a bit.)

Try to take your Morning Brainiac's Energizing Cocktail upon waking on an empty stomach. You'll want to wait about 40+ minutes before having your first 10-Hour Coffee Diet coffee to give the supplements a chance to absorb and get their full effects.

I realize you might never have heard of some of these supplements before. I'll cover each of them and where you can get them before the chapter ends.

An Optional Afternoon Second Dose

The Morning Brainiac's Energizing Cocktail is powerful and will do wonders.

You *can* take a second helping. I'd take just the first for a week or so, especially if you're female, and see how things go. If you feel great and see results in your body through the supplements and the brain-healthy foods you're now eating, then you have to decide if a second cocktail would be a waste or if it would multiply the good that is already happening. And if you try it, you might want to return to just one due to expense or due to the fact that you don't notice added benefits from two helpings. (I won't be surprised if one is all you want or need... one does wonders.)

If you do take a second helping or just want to see how it goes with an additional dose, wait until the mid or late afternoon and have it away from your 10-Hour Coffee Diet coffee or meal.

The Bedtime Brainiac's Sleepy-time Cocktail

Your brain can work on your body best when you get out of the way! One way to do so is to take the Bedtime Brainiac's Sleepy-time Cocktail right before bedtime to boost your Fantastic Four chemical nutrients and work on your body as a result.

Before you go to bed, take this:

- One and a half teaspoons of GABA
- Three, and perhaps six to nine grams of Melatonin (details about dosage for Melatonin and the other supplements will follow below)
- 200 mg of 5-HTP
- 400-600 mg of Magnesium

Note: Don't drink green tea or any other caffeine with your Bedtime Brainiac's Sleepy-time Cocktail. Take with pure, filtered, chlorine-free water.

With melatonin you may want to begin with three grams and see how you do. In a small number of people, 3 grams of melatonin helps them sleep, but an added amount actually wakes them up in the middle of the night.

I brush my teeth before bed and I always take my Bedtime Brainiac's Sleepy-time Cocktail a few minutes *before* I brush my teeth and rinse my mouth. This gives the supplements a chance to clear my esophagus and begin working before I go to bed.

A Look at the Specifics

If want you to know more about each of the supplements, I listed the specifics for you below.

L-Tyrosine

L-Tyrosine boosts dopamine production. It's an amino acid that forms a protein building block in your body. You get L-Tyrosine naturally from meat and dairy sources as well as nuts and quality wheat and oats. The supplement speeds up your quantity and builds up your dopamine levels more rapidly than through food alone. Your energy and focus should increase through your building up of L-Tyrosine.

If you're in the USA you can purchase L-Tyrosine capsules through Amazon.com or Bodybuilding.com. My favorite brand is the *NOW* brand.

Here is a link to it on Amazon: amazon.com/NOW-Foods-L-Tyrosine-500mg-120cap/dp/B000ELR896

Note: I suggest that you purchase two or three bottles of 120 capsules. One bottle at the recommended doses of 3 grams a day would last no longer than 20 days (around 6 capsules a day at the minimum) so you need to purchase multiple bottles when you buy it.

L-Tyrosine is the single most important brain supplement that I think you *must* take when you begin to restore and energize your brain and body. For the average person, 30 days minimum is ideal to get the brain properly optimized for weight loss.

Whether I take the Morning Brainiac's Energizing Cocktail or not, I always take L-Tyrosine daily (except for the once in a while when I forget) to help maintain proper brain health, reduce cravings and appetite, increase energy levels, lower stress levels, and enhance mood. Once you take it and notice a difference you'll probably not want to stop taking it after the initial 30-60 day trial period.

St. John's Wort

St. John's Wort is known to be an anti-depression herb. Other problems related to depression such as anxiety, tiredness, and insomnia can be helped through St. John's Wort.

You can take 300 mg twice daily. St. John's Wort will help boost serotonin levels. Amazingly, it has been shown to ease symptoms of OCD in some individuals who suffer with that.

You can get St. John's Wort on Amazon at this link: amazon.com/Foods-JohnS-Wort-300Mg-Capsulesc /dp/B0013OSSBA/

L-Phenylalanine

L-Phenylalanine, like L-Tyrosine, is a protein building block known as an amino acid. You can get L-Phenylalanine through meat and dairy and eggs.

You can take L-Phenylalanine twice daily. L-Phenylalanine promotes dopamine in your body and can improve your mental acumen and alertness.

You can get L-Phenylalanine here: amazon.com/NOW-Foods-L-Phenylalanine-500mg-Capsules/dp/B000JCN2MW

Note: For hypertension patients, L-Phenylalanine can increase blood pressure. Although hypertension patients aren't warned to stay away from L-Phenylalanine, after all it is a naturally occurring amino acid, if you take the supplement you should monitor your blood pressure regularly to ensure your BP doesn't increase due to the L-Phenylalanine. But of course, if you're a hypertension patient you should be monitoring your blood pressure regularly anyway. Home blood pressure kits are highly accurate and simple to use, especially those made by *Omron*.

Note: Cancer patients are encouraged to avoid L-Phenylalanine.

DMAE

DMAE is basically the B vitamin called choline. DMAE strongly influences your production of acetylcholine and by adding DMAE you in effect add to your acetylcholine reserve. DMAE produces age-lowering effects, helps with aggression, and improves mental ability in our memory stores.

You can get DMAE here: amazon.com/Twinlab-DMAE-Caps-100-capsules/dp/B000RZ943M/

Acetyl Carnitine (ALCAR)

Acetyl Carnitine, aka Acetyl-L-Carnitine, aka ALCAR is another amino acid protein building block. ALCAR works as an antioxidant and keeps your cells from aging as rapidly as they otherwise might. This keeps your brain cells young as long as possible. ALCAR also is used to treat neuro-related problems such as Parkinson's. ALCAR's amazing properties crosses the brain line and even have shown to improve male fertility. Your heart, brain, and muscles all appear to benefit from ALCAR, perhaps a process of ALCAR causing your cells to communicate better through reduced inflammation. You can take ALCAR with the morning cocktail or right before you exercise.

You can get ALCAR here: amazon.com/Foods-Acetyl-L-Carnitine-500mg-Vcaps/dp/B000QSLINE/

Lecithin Granules (acetylcholine)

Lecithin granules improve your nervous system, breathing, and boost your energy levels. About a third of your brain is composed of lecithin with lots of lecithin appearing on your myelin insulators throughout your brain.

You can get Lecithin granules here (be sure to get the Non-GMO): amazon.com/Lecithin-Granules-Non-GMO-1-Pounds/dp/B0001TRQY8/

B-12

B-12 deficiency can show itself as a nervous system malady and anemia problems. Almost any meat or fish (including shellfish) or dairy and eggs will have B-12. Sometimes certain people's stomachs don't absorb B-12 properly which can cause problems, but a healthy diet will provide adequate B-12 and supplements just ensures that even more.

Strict vegans don't get B-12 in their diets and must take supplements. (They also don't get enough protein through their food sources to have healthy brains.) In eating the right kinds of low-carb, high-protein food as well as supplementing with B-12 you'll feel better and improve the odds you have a healthy nervous system.

You can get B-12 here: amazon.com/Twin-Lab-B-12-Dots-250-Count/dp/B003WLQLBQ/

Yohimbine HCL

The first of the two optional ingredients in the Morning Brainiac's Energizing Cocktail is Yohimbine HCL. Yohimbine HCL helps promote fat loss and has been shown to help men's sexual dysfunction problems. Yohimbine HCL has been used to aid in the treatment of memory problems as well.

Take only 2.5mg and make sure it says Yohimbine HCL and not Yohimbe. Also make sure it says HCL.

You can purchase Yohimbine HCL here: amazon.com/Yohimbine-2-5-HCL-2-5g/dp/B0041N2F9Q/

GABA

Yes, you can add GABA directly to your body and brain.

Taking too much GABA makes you sedated and too little causes the problems mentioned earlier in the book. Given that GABA can work as a sedation chemical makes it a great supplement to use at bedtime.

One and a half teaspoons (suggested for your Bedtime Brainiac's Sleepy-time Cocktail) is about two and a half grams of GABA.

You can get GABA here: amazon.com/NOW-Foods-Gaba-750mg-Vcaps/dp/B0013OVZAG

With the pill, you'll take three to four of the 750 mg pills before bed. The bottle lasts about 30 days or so at the recommended dosage.

Melatonin

Melatonin is a hormone that regulates sleep and your body naturally produces it. As a supplement, people take anywhere from three to nine milligrams of melatonin before bed. As you saw earlier, it's a great addition to your Bedtime Brainiac's Sleepy-time Cocktail. If you see results with three milligrams, meaning you sleep well throughout the night, stick with three. If you want a little extra help, try six and then nine milligrams.

When you reach a good dose for you, you will often find that you sleep extremely well and wake up refreshed.

From Amazon you can get melatonin here: amazon.com/Nature-Made-Melatonin-Tablets-Value/dp

/B005DEK990/

5-HTP

5-HTP, also known as 5-Hydroxytryptophan, is a by-product of the protein building block L-tryptophan. 5-HTP can help your nervous system and brain and your overall feeling and attitude by helping you produce more serotonin. That is why 5-HTP is used a lot for depression when antidepressants fail (as they often do). Also, 5-HTP is great for encouraging weight loss due to the serotonin producing a natural, "up" emotional state so we don't reach for food to comfort us as much as before.

For 5-HTP, I suggest you get the *NOW* brand that has 100 mg per capsules and 120 capsules per bottle.

Here is the link to 5-HTP on Amazon's site: amazon.com/NOW-Foods-5-HTP-100mg-VCaps/dp/B0013OQI1W/

Magnesium

Magnesium helps regulate the heart, can help adjust blood pressure, and helps alleviate brittleness that can attack bones. Although severe magnesium deficiencies are rare, almost everyone is deficient in magnesium to some degree.

For most of us, magnesium helps keep us from wanting to "graze" constantly on food because we're less anxious and feel more focused. Magnesium is a sleep aid as well. Our brains love magnesium because it helps encourage the production of GABA.

Spinach and kale are great sources of magnesium.

You can get magnesium from Amazon here: amazon.com/Doctors-Best-Absorption-Magnesium-Elemental/dp/B000BD0RT0/

Additional Supplements You Might Find Useful

I'd like to suggest just a few more supplements that anyone who wants a better brain and body may find useful.

Liquid Cod Liver Oil

Hundreds of thousands of great-grandmothers can't all be wrong and one of their favorite health tricks was to feed all the children in the household cod liver oil. They didn't care about the science behind it. They only knew that it kept away all sorts of problems. And in our modern world it still does, if not more so.

You'll get beneficial omega-3 oil and improve your brain and body's lubrication and more. Acetylcholine production seems to be boosted by cod liver oil. It works as a wonderful essential fatty acid and you can get cod living oil in liquid form here: bodybuilding.com/store/tl/codoil.html and here: amazon.com/TwinLab-Norwegian-Liver-Plain-liquid/dp/B00012TQPW/

> **Note:** Cod liver oil, as well as other fat supplements you might take, should be taken with food for the highest benefit... or with your 10-Hour Coffee Diet coffee. A good time is immediately following a meal. About one gram with each meal will keep your omega-3 up and your brain working more smoothly. For the above liquid cod liver oil, I suggest 1 teaspoon with each meal.

Not everybody can handle taking cod liver oil in liquid form but I suggest you do so if you can. If you find it difficult to take in liquid form you can consume either fish oil pills or cod liver oil pills.

Cod Liver Oil or Fish Oil Pills

I don't recommend getting cod liver oil in pill form because it's not economical and you'll have to take too many pills with each meal. But if you need to take this supplement in pill form, here you go:

amazon.com/Nature-Made-Omega-3-1200mg-Softgels/dp/B0026RHHEW/

Chromium Picolinate

Chromium Picolinate is an old standby supplement for bodybuilders and anyone else who wants to fight flab. Chromium Picolinate is a trace mineral that you can get from food, but to help with fat loss and recover quicker from workouts, 200 mcg (*not* mg) will work nicely for you taken once daily with a meal.

You can get Chromium Picolinate from Amazon here: amazon.com/Foods-Chromium-Picolinate-200mcg-Capsules/dp/B0019LPNLK/

Your Brain and Sleep – Quality Trumps Quantity but Both are Critical

We've covered quite a bit about sleep already.

By taking the Bedtime Brainiac's Sleepy-time Cocktail, your sleep time should become one that you don't notice except in the morning when you awaken and feel incredibly refreshed. Sleep should no longer be something that comes only after tossing and turning. Waking in the middle of the night for long stretches of time should be a thing of the past.

When we sleep well, our bodies repair damage done from movement and toxins we acquired previously. Our bodies can digest whatever food remains in our system and grab nutrients from our food and supplements more easily than when we're awake. Dreaming allows our minds to straighten up and remove baggage.

> **Note:** The production of good cholesterol seems to occur more at night during sleep than in the daytime. This is why people with high levels of bad cholesterol (LDL) often find that supplementing with 20 mgs or so of Policosanol before bedtime can lower LDL whereas taken at other times will have less of an effect. If you tend to have higher LDL you might consider adding 20 mgs to your Bedtime Brainiac's Sleepy-time Cocktail.

Sleep Issues Resolved

Those with low GABA levels find their sleep interrupted and restless. That is why the Bedtime Brainiac's Sleepy-time Cocktail includes GABA as a direct supplement. As you learned in the previous chapter, melatonin also works to help you get to sleep and stay that way.

The less you sleep the more stress your body has to combat. Sleep is a cure for normal stress. Even if you get a "full night's sleep," if the sleep was restless, then you'll awaken in the morning groggy, cranky, and completely unrested. Your stress level will be high and remain that way which burns out your dopamine faster, as well as acetylcholine and serotonin. This is why working on improving all four of your brain's nutrient chemicals is so critical; a decrease in one can cause problems in the other. It's best to boost all of them.

You Might Try This

Lots of factors go into a good night's sleep besides what you've consumed and your supplement levels.

Some people can sleep through anything and sleep hard while doing so. But for most of us, especially as we age, sleep doesn't come as easily as it did when our bodies were young.

Balancing your brain's dopamine, serotonin, GABA, and acetylcholine is perhaps the number one thing you can do to get a better night's sleep. But if you're diligently working to balance your brain and body, and you're using the supplements, but you still have a few sleep issues, it would be helpful to rule out environmental causes of sleep disorders before going any further. Many factors outside our bodies affect our sleep habits and patterns.

Here are some tips that have been found to help people sleep more soundly:

- Sleep in an all-dark room. This means no lights, not even nightlights. This means turn your digital alarm clock's display down to its lowest brightness level, if it has one, and face it away from you. This means getting shades for all windows so that outside lights won't wake your mind. See, our bodies are designed to begin waking us up when it starts to get lighter. That may be all well and good, but today's modern age puts unnatural light all around us even at night. Sometimes our spouses want a light kept on so they don't trip in the middle of the night and often they may want to read long after we want to sleep. If you can't darken the room to your satisfaction, get an eye mask to block out light.

- During the day do the opposite! Get out in the sun if it's a nice day. If you work indoors, go out at lunch and on breaks. The sun and fresh outdoor air revives you during your waking hours and actually prepares your body for sleep later when it gets dark.
- Keep noise away from you. This is often difficult if you live in a busy city, in a dorm, or in an apartment. Earplugs will keep the noise out. Some people do not do well with earplugs because the plugs stop up the ears and that can be bothersome. If the noise isn't too great, try putting cotton in your ears. This muffles noise without giving you that stopped-up feeling. If nothing else works, "white noise" will often drown out any noise problems. Find static that is consistent and not going in and out. I personally use a Sleep Mate white noise machine I bought from Amazon.com. This is an example of "white noise" which means a specific, steady noise without any spikes in the sound.
- Remove the TV from your bedroom. Make your bedroom a place for sleep (and fun) and leave lesser forms of entertainment like television in another part of the house. Television wakes up your mind right when you need to be letting your mind rev down for the evening.
- If your mate insists on a TV or MP3 player or radio before they go to sleep (some people do better with them than without them), it's only fair if they use earphones. You can find lots of wireless headphone options for television online and at department stores.
- Reading works wonders or wakes people up depending on their own make-up. If you're one who goes to sleep easily after reading a few pages, by all means make that a habit. If not, stop taking your books to bed with you. If you read on a Kindle or other eBook reader, the focused bright light sometimes will awaken you more than if you read a regular book or kept a lamp on next to you. So if you read eBooks in bed to sleep, you'll usually find that leaving a lamp on at the same time enables you to get sleepier faster than if you didn't leave the side light on in spite of the fact that this would seem to be the opposite of reality.
- Don't take your laptop to bed for the same reasons as the previous two tips.
- Do what you can to develop a regular sleep schedule. Your body likes habits. If your schedule allows it, you should attempt to get to bed and get up at the same time every day. Taking the weekend off to sleep in doesn't do you any good; it can easily make you feel worse and get less restful sleep the other days. As long as you're sleeping well throughout the night five nights a week you will feel far better if you continue doing so on the weekends too.
- Keep your room as cool as you can stand. Our sleep is a lot like a mini hibernation for the winter. Although it's difficult to sleep when we're too cold, a cool room improves your body's desire to drift off.
- Eat turkey; the tryptophan increases your serotonin, which makes you happy and more oblivious to problems of the outside world. Some warm milk will also help as long as it's raw, whole milk where the lactose sugar hasn't been processed enough to disturb your energy level as is the case with the dreaded homogenized and pasteurized kind that most stores sell.

This sure sounds like a lot of work to sleep, doesn't it?

Well, you don't have to implement every one of these tonight. If you're having trouble sleeping even after taking your brain's supplements for a couple of weeks, you probably have a general idea of what the trouble might be, such as your room not being dark enough. Work on the most obvious solutions first. Then try lowering the temperature if that doesn't work. Then try the rest of the tips if you need more. You'll eventually find yourself not realizing you've drifted off until you wake the next morning feeling great and refreshed.

Your Brain and Sex – Quality *and* Quantity Are Signs of a Youthful Brain No Matter What Your Physical Age Is

Fix your brain and you'll have better sex!

When it gets better, you'll usually have more of it too.

As people age, we generally think of them as having less sex. We think that because it's true. Generally speaking, starting in our 30's or slightly before we begin to want sex less even if our drive was previously higher than normal. It's relative, but we do slow down in the physical pleasure department as we get older for a number of reasons.

Work and family issues will begin to consume time we used to spend in bed with our partners. Physical changes such as weight gain, relationship conflicts (which may be increased because one or both of you have some serotonin and dopamine levels out of whack!), lower levels of testosterone and estrogen hormones, a slowing down of our metabolism that results in a desire to do less physical movement overall, and scores of other factors can determine how much our sex drive and activities decrease.

Slowing Down Your Slowdown

You can slow the slowing down. That means you can increase the amount of sex that you have, but more importantly you can increase the amount you actually want by fixing your brain and body. You may not go back to the four times daily from your Honeymoon, but you can go back a decade or two (age dependent). Sex is the intimate activity that you and your partner share that is not available to others and it's critical that you keep that special bond that only the two of you (are supposed to) share.

You can help improve and even save your relationship when the two of you are eager to share this special togetherness. Even if you're not concerned about a lower sex drive, you should welcome the chance to be happier in your relationship because many other relationship problems can dissolve. Sex won't solve major conflicts, but it can bring you closer.

And it's fun. And it feels good. It's win-win for both of you if you can boost your sex drive together through boosting your brain.

Your Brain and Body's Love Connection to Overall Health

As I'll explain with exercise in the next chapter, there is a synergy between your brain and sex. A healthy sex life encourages a healthy brain and body. A healthy brain and body encourages a healthy sex life. All three, your brain, body, and sexual passion work together to help the others.

For men who have heart trouble, the first question often asked is, "Can I still have sex?" Surprisingly, the answer is almost always "yes" with a few initial precautions. So a man might not be able to return to work after a heart attack for a long period of time, but he can resume making love to his partner in fairly quick order, in spite of the fact that we view the latter as being more physical.

The truth is that making love more often can help *reduce* the risks related to strokes and heart attacks in men. Plus, prostate problems are often warded off and can even disappear in their early stages when more sex is enjoyed more often.

Speaking of men, in general men can gain a tremendous number of benefits from putting their bodies and brains into proper balance. Erectile dysfunction, impotence, and a lack of desire in both men and women can be corrected through diet and exercise in many cases. Think about serotonin and dopamine, the "Happy" and "Reward" brain chemicals. More of them make us happy and feel rewarded and when we're happy and confident our sex drive will improve almost instantly. Depressed patients hardly ever think of sex and the very idea will drive many of them even deeper into their funk.

With women the advantages are even more! Menstrual cycles can become more regular with regular sex. Your periods can be less troublesome and lighter. Your moods are better and you'll find it easier to keep weight off and maintain muscle tone. This all works together to help keep your immune system strong to avoid colds and flus.

Stress and sex go together like oil and water. Your stress is reduced when your brain is in balance. It's no secret that stress is a barrier for women to want sex. For men, stress is often a *reason* to have sex in hopes he can relax. This opposite reaction to stress in men and women can cause all kinds of problems when both are stressed. Reducing the stress through a balanced GABA and serotonin helps make that conflict disappear.

Food, Spice, and Spicier Sex

The foods that you are beginning to eat to help your brain function better will also directly help your sex life. Through the higher protein your muscles will strengthen, your bones will begin to lose some brittleness that may be creeping into them, and your body will become more limber and, for lack of better term, "juicier" through the vegetables and more pure water that you now are encouraged to consume. (And on second thought, "juicier" is probably the best term possible in this case.)

Fibrous and leafy and colorful vegetables will improve your circulation and make your hormone production far more beneficial and normal. So will the eating of protein-rich meats and eggs. Some vegetables improve your pheromones, the odors you omit that usually are beneath our conscious radar that attracts the opposite sex.

Lowered desire for fast food and a higher consumption of good fats such as nuts create bodies ripe for sex. Selenium from Brazil nuts is great for increasing your sexual appetite. Almonds seem to give men a testosterone boost.

Spices such as cayenne pepper will increase your metabolism. Your nerve endings will become more sensitive which is a sex booster. Garlic increases blood flow and other spices will boost your desire for lovemaking.

Supplements for Sex

While an entire book can be written on supplements and improved sexual desire and performance, it's surprising how little many of us have to do in order to greatly improve our sexual function and desire.

I'd like to discuss just a few supplements that improve sexual well-being. Fortunately, some of these ways you'll already be using as you fix your brain! For example, fish oil will do wonders for mood and will keep your joints lubricated ensuring that you are more limber when you and your partner start fooling around. Muscle and joint soreness and stiffness act against a happy physical union and without those troubles you will both enjoy your sessions far more.

5-HTP

The 5-HTP seems to help some women relax enough to focus on and enjoy sex far more. Generally speaking, women are strongly emotional and being able to turn off our emotions from a hectic workday or from some problem around the house is difficult. What our minds know but our emotions won't allow sometimes is that good sex can free us from some of the emotional troubles of the world but it's those troubles that keep us from enjoying sex to begin with.

The vicious cycle can be helped through the brain supplements. 5-HTP is a good one for those who might be experiencing emotional barriers to being able to focus on sex with their partner.

DHEA

DHEA converts to a sexual hormone and also helps balance our weight issues. Surprisingly, DHEA is one of the most abundant hormones in the body and yet little is said about DHEA.

Getting a DHEA supplement, especially a high quality one through a homeopath-based medical doctor, can not only enhance your sex life and keep your waistline down. Your dopamine levels will benefit from increased DHEA, creating a happier and more vibrant relationship between you and others.

DHEA is one supplement you should get some medical advice for, again through a homeopath-based medical doctor if possible. Some health issues such as current and former cancer patients, as well as pregnant and nursing mothers need to have approval before getting DHEA although fortunately alternatives for them are sometimes available.

SAMe

SAMe, also known as S-adenosyl-methionine, helps in the production of dopamine, serotonin, and other brain transmitting chemicals. You naturally produce melatonin, and hence probably sleep well, if you have ample supply of SAMe. For our needs here, SAMe also helps give you an energy boost before and during sex and enables you to be more passionate with your mate.

A Natural Viagra for Men

Five mgs of yohimbine HCL and four to six grams of citrulline malate each day will begin to reduce erectile problems in many men. Stop worrying about Viagra. Heck, just stop worrying at all and try this combo out. Two and a half milligrams of yohimbine HCL and two or three grams of citrulline malate twice daily will improve the sexual performance of many men who try it, once again trumping expensive and risky drugs that mask symptoms instead of solving problems.

Ideally you should take these in two doses on an empty stomach during the day, especially on days you are planning a sexual escapade. Try your best to take one of the doses within two hours of going to bed or two hours before having sex.

Citrulline malate is a precursor to arginine, which improves circulation and the travel of nitric oxide to the penis. Citrulline is actually better for men's sexual organ health than arginine supplementation, which is often suggested; arginine is simply not a better supplement in most cases.

We already provided you with a link to yohimbine HCl previously. Here is where you can get citrulline malate: amazon.com/PRIMAFORCE-Citrulline-Malate-200-Grams/dp/B002JIO4R6/

Exercise to Take Years off Your Brain and Enhance Your Mind's Horsepower

You don't fix your brain so you can exercise more. You exercise more to fix your brain.

Your brain's balance is needed before your body goes into balance. You know that already. But one thing to do to help get your brain's nutrients boosted and balanced is to exercise. Fortunately, the quality of exercise is more important to helping your brain than the quantity. For now you should work on making the most of each workout, maximizing your brain's activity along the way.

Once your brain is on board and functioning like a lean, mean exercising machine, your brain will begin to turn on switches in your body to boost your exercise performance and improve your results. This brain/body synergy is a wonderful thing to experience because you are physically and emotionally encouraged to do more and not make excuses as we are all prone to do when we don't feel motivated due to a sluggish brain.

Calorie Restrictive Diets Restrict Exercise

One reason calorie restrictive diets fail is that a person gets so hungry they begin to crave food in a way that they simply cannot control and they go on a binge. This binging is your body's way of fighting starvation. Your body wants to store food in case the starvation returns any time soon.

Another reason starvation diets are so bad for us is they limit exercise. You simply don't have the fuel to exercise and when you force yourself to do it your movements will not be productive enough to make a big difference.

One of the benefits of a plan such as the 10-Hour Coffee Diet and other low-carb diets is that high protein and high fat foods keep your body from wanting to pack on fat. Your cravings for the bad stuff stay at bay. You will have more energy even though having a lot of eggs and turkey at breakfast the first few days looks like it might put you in a deep sleep for the next 2 weeks. The reality is that it does the opposite, giving you more energy and allowing you to build and repair muscles that wouldn't be feasible under a higher-carb diet plan and would be impossible under a calorie restrictive diet.

> **Note:** Stay hydrated during any exercise, whether you're performing cardio or resistance training. If you sweat a lot you'll want to add some extra sea salt in your next meal to replace the needed sodium balance you will lose through exercise. In addition, the loss of all that fast food you used to eat means you'll have

a lower amount of sodium in your system to begin with so as a general rule, whether you have exercised heavily or not, you should add salt to your low-carb foods... enough to taste, but not enough to overpower the food. Remember, much of your taste will come from the delicious brain-healthy spices you are now using so look at salt more of a supplement that you need to keep your sodium level in good shape and not use salt for a primary flavoring as much as you may have done before.

Maximize Your Exercise Through Timing

Again, in this short chapter on your brain/body connection to exercise, I want to show you ways to be more effective with less time and effort. One of the ways to do that with exercise is to time it properly.

One of the best bits of advice I can give you in one paragraph is that when you exercise in the morning you will raise your metabolism throughout the rest of the day. That means that you have longer in the day to burn more calories and be more energetic when you need that energy to work and accomplish what life requires.

The Fantastic Four and Exercise

Your four brain chemicals just delight in your exercise!

Consider these points:

- Exercise stimulates dopamine production.
- Aerobic exercise can restore acetylcholine levels.
- GABA is improved through Pilates and other forms of aerobic relaxation.
- Serotonin will exhibit itself more through just about *any* movement. Too many people harm their serotonin levels by sitting all day at a desk job. You don't have to go all out to reverse this problem. Just get up throughout the day, even when you don't need a break. Smart phone apps and computer utility programs are available for free that provide timers. Set your timer for 50 minutes of work and when the timer dings, you walk around the office a bit, get a drink of fresh, clean water to lubricate your system, and perhaps have four or five almonds to ward off hunger.

For the nighttime, you'll want to begin to slow your body down. Even if a passionate night with your partner is in the works, slowing down after work to free your mind and relax your body will preserve some needed energy for later when you get to bed. After dinner, take a walk. The fresh air is an underutilized pick-me-up in today's air-conditioned/heated world. Praying, chanting, singing, and humming also can help slow your mind down and get the toxins of cares and worries out of your system.

Yes, winding down is as important a part of your physical life as exercise.

Exercise Makes You Young

Exercise benefits are so numerous and obvious that I feel silly even list some of them...

- You are more limber
- You feel better
- You have less fat
- Your skin is more pliable
- Your bones are stronger
- You sleep better
- You ward off severe heart and lung and blood sugar diseases
- You will desire more sex
- Your body utilized oxygen more efficiently so cells communicate better
- Your body builds more brain cells
- You will think more clearly

- Your body gets faster
- Your reflexes become more responsive
- You have less tendency to be depressed or anxious
- Your ward off the aging effects of Alzheimer's and other memory-related diseases

In other words, you become younger when you exercise.

The only thing that doesn't get younger is your actual age, but otherwise every aspect of you gets younger.

All of those younger attributes appear when you begin to boost your Fantastic Four brain chemicals through supplements also.

In other words, focusing on your brain and body gives you a three-fold attack on aging. In many ways you can get younger a lot faster by starting with your brain instead of focusing on diet or exercise alone as we've been doing for most of the recent past.

The Traditional Lies of Resistance and Aerobics

You should focus both on cardio as well as resistance training. For some reason, women have often been made to think that they should stay away from strength training or they will produce man-like bulging, unsightly muscles. Hogwash!

Lean and limber is the result of women doing routine resistance training. Toning your muscles means that your metabolism will burn faster and your body will utilize the food you eat as fuel and not try to store it as flab.

Don't believe the lie that an hour or two of aerobics means an incredible you. That falsehood has caused a lot of exercise-related problems over the past few decades, the worst of which have even resulted in early graves. Our bodies have developed through time to be tested with a heavy, fast, and high-energy state, but only for short periods of time.

Do you ever watch the Olympics? Think about this. The first time I learned about what I'm about to tell you, I was blown away by the truth that has stared at us in the face every four years at the Olympics and yet we still believe that tons of aerobics are good for us. We still feel guilty that we don't do aerobics more or stick with them when we do start going to a spinning class.

Here it is: What do the Olympic long-distance runners look like? Lanky, tall, thin, bags of bones, right? And there's a reason. To run such long distances and not cause cardiac arrest by the time they're 16 their bodies must shed all muscle mass and become little more than hollow shells.

Now, have you ever noticed what the sprinting competitors look like?

They all seem to have nice, full chests, great backs, great legs, muscular, not a speck of fat, confident, they don't have that constant far-away look in their eyes, they smile a lot, and watch them interact with others and you'll see they laugh and joke with their team members and coaches (grumpy long distance runners never seem to do this much).

Wonder why?

I am certain we know why. Our bodies are designed to handle brief moments of stress. That is how we can escape danger. That is how we can express emotion instantly. That is how we catch a glass that we bump off a table (sometimes we catch it!). We're designed to handle everyday things.

Our bodies are made for sprinting and not for aerobics.

Do you want to look as unhealthy as most long-distance runner you've seen? Even if it means you can run 5 miles without stopping? Or do you want that amazing, perfectly proportioned body that we develop through work-rest-work-rest activity?

You can spend two hours at the gym each day doing aerobics and getting thin and mean (as opposed to lean and mean, very different vernaculars here!) or you can perform interval kinds of training like sprints, do a couple of days or resistance training, and spend far less time exercising, get far better results, and have a healthy brain and a good-looking body.

Look, I know some of you reading this do long-distance jogging. Please don't take my criticisms of it personally. If long-distance jogging is enjoyable and works for you, consider yourself lucky. But for most everyone else there are better exercise options.

14

BRAIN SUMMARY

So there you have it.

Fix your brain and fix your body. It works that way best. You'll rarely do your brain much good if you work on your body first. You will be working against yourself, going against the grain or pushing a boulder uphill to use analogous phrases.

Fix your brain first and your brain will then *help you* fix your body.

We've presented you with a lot of options in this section. The core thing to remember is that if you are having problems losing weight and feeling energetic even though you "eat good" and exercise a lot, then maybe diet and exercise aren't the most important problems holding you back from losing weight and feeling great.

Maybe the problem is a brain that is unbalanced.

Our advice is simple. Incorporate the diet and exercise advice in this book, but concentrate on fixing your brain for the next month or two. With a balanced and healthy brain, exercise and diet will have an easier time helping you to lose weight.

We've mentioned a bunch of supplements and yes they do cost money. Better quality foods suggested in this book also tend to cost more money too. There is no getting around that. However, if you improve your brain by following the 10-Hour Coffee Diet advice, you may not even need to buy most or all of the supplements listed. I already broke down the food cost savings by following the diet. $200+ a month!

I'm sure your health, how you look, and how you feel are important to you or you wouldn't be reading this book. For various reasons people around the world are becoming fatter and unhealthier with each passing year. The medical costs associated with that are expensive. Even if the diet and supplements did cost you more than you're currently paying for food and supplements, why not pay a little bit more now for truly healthy foods and supplements and in the meantime live a higher quality life rather than spending more later on medical bills while dragging on through life with too many pounds and too little energy?

Section 3

–

All the Other Good Stuff

15

DIGGING DEEPER INTO COCONUT OIL –HOW TO USE COCONUT OIL TO LOSE WEIGHT, RADICALLY IMPROVE YOUR HEALTH AND ENERGY LEVELS, AND BECOME MORE ATTRACTIVE

As you now know, one of the 3 Weird Tricks of the 10-Hour Coffee Diet is extra virgin coconut oil.

This marvelously healthy fat is such a workhorse of health that it deserves its own separate chapter in this book. Here, you won't get a review of the diet. That's been covered. You will learn all sorts of other benefits that you didn't see earlier as well as learn the uses that make this one of the most versatile items in the kitchen.

Let me repeat a few benefits that were mentioned earlier:

- Smaller waistlines
- More energy
- Better-tasting meals
- Healthier hair and skin
- Cleaner and therefore healthier teeth[56]
- Retards and can even reverse Alzheimer's, Parkinson's, and ALS[57]
- Improves Type 1 and Type 2 diabetes[58]

- Improves or heals several skin conditions including fungal infections, acne, eczema, psoriasis, and rosacea[59]
- Kills candida fungus[60]
- Kills many bacteria *and* viruses
- Can retard, reduce, and even help reverse autism[61]

We'll Keep it Short and Simple

I want to tell you the "what" and "why" of coconut oil. I want to excite you about coconut oil because I believe in it and I wouldn't be doing you justice if I didn't do my best to convince you to add it into your family's lifelong eating plan.

I'm opinionated, but that means I tell you what I've learned and you can make up your own mind. For example, I almost always tell people about coconut oil's benefits any time the topic of diet or health arises.

I'm a Coconut Oil Fanatic– Not Everybody Is

Coconut oil has properties that will surprise you. Almost all of its properties are benefits. Actually, I know of *no* anti-benefits as long as you use a high-quality, organic coconut oil.

Given how good it is, it's not surprising that it's been maligned as well. One of the most famous examples happened in the 1990s. The CSPI, *Center for Science in the Public Interest* – one of the most misnamed groups ever formed – said cooking popcorn in coconut oil is unhealthy.[62] Yes, they made national headline news with their unfounded announcement that this perfectly natural, health-promoting fat is unhealthy.

While nothing could be further from the truth, they went on to compound damage to those who listened to them. The CSPI made it clear that *popcorn* is healthy, but cooking the popcorn in coconut oil made the popcorn unhealthy.

That is sort of bonkers! Some might even say that is borderline fraudulent at best and life-damaging at worst.

Humans were not created to digest grains in mass quantities, and we especially get too much corn in our diets. From the dangerous High Fructose Corn Syrup found in almost every pre-packaged product on the market to the genetically-modified corn that provides the bulk found in almost every product sold on store shelves, we're drowning in corn. Our health (and waistlines) shows the result.

I've already discussed how grains often affect us negatively and how fats such as coconut oils affect us positively. For now, it's intriguing that the product that is bad for us in quantity – popcorn – is not maligned and one of the only healthy things about some popcorn – the coconut oil it's popped in – is given the boot.

Good Fat is Good for You!

To put your weight (and health) into high efficient gear, you need to eat more fat. Yes, this goes against everything that's been touted for about four decades.

Fat should comprise at least 30 to 35% of your diet. The healthy fat you need comes from source such as healthy oils like coconut and olive oil, organic seeds, grass-fed butter, raw milk, organic eggs, and nuts.

It's not that fats are good for you; it's that *good* fats are good for you.

There is a huge difference between manufactured fats, naturally occurring bad fats, and naturally occurring healthy fats.

Back to Coconut Oil

I need to get back to the specifics of coconut oil. Still, it was required that I show strong evidence for why good fats are good for you. I'll also demonstrate that more fats *help you lose weight*. Fat in your diet does *not* translate to fat on your thighs.

Can I leave you with one remaining item? It is just something scientifically verified by an independent source. The low-fat diet craze moved into the mainstream in the 1970s by the McGovern Committee. It has contributed to a major boom in diseases such as Alzheimer's. *Lack of good fats* gives such diseases a better foothold.

You can click to see the footnote for the source. The title of the article is so telling: *Coconut Oil and Alzheimer's: Is the Low-Fat Diet and Cholesterol-Lowering Drugs Part of the Problem?*[63]

Let's Get This Over With Now – Buy *This* Coconut Oil If Possible

I know that the number one question will be, "What kind of coconut oil should I get?"

In the 10-Hour Coffee Diet, you had a lot to process. In addition, there were several items you needed to get before you could even begin the plan. I mentioned a low-cost extra-virgin olive oil to get you going. If that's all you ever use, you'll be fine. No, you'll be *much better off* than if you didn't add ample coconut oil into you and your family's diet.

But I want to tell you about the very *best* coconut oil money can buy. If times are tight, just file this away for later. You can always upgrade to this better oil.

The short answer is that you should only get a coconut oil that meets all these conditions:

- Is an *organic* coconut oil
- Is a *virgin* coconut oil
- Is cold-pressed

If you stick with those three requirements, you will be buying better coconut oil for you and your family than 99% of all other coconut oil buyers.

Virgin – Taste and Quality

When oil such as coconut oil or olive oil is labeled as "virgin," it means that independent labs extensively tested it to ensure quality and flavor.[64] In addition, the virgin label helps ensure that original product – olives for example, or the coconuts used to extract the oil – are pure, not created through strange cross-pollination experimentation, and that no additives were added during the creation process to affect the taste or freshness or quality in any way.

When it comes to coconut oil, there is no industry standard for the terms "virgin" or "extra virgin" as there is with olive oil. So a product labeled "extra virgin" coconut oil doesn't necessarily mean much over a similar product labeled "virgin" coconut oil. The first organization to attempt to standardize "virgin" coconut oil was Tropical Traditions. (You will soon see that I am big on that company.)

If a coconut oil producer states that they follow the Tropical Traditions guidelines, you know the following:

> They used only fresh coconut meat or what is called *non-copra.* Chemicals and high heating are not used in further refining, since the natural, pure coconut oil is very stable with a shelf life of several years. There are currently two main processes of manufacturing Virgin Coconut Oil:
>
> 1. Quick drying of fresh coconut meat, which is then used to press out the oil. Using this method, the coconut meat is quick dried, and the oil is then pressed out via mechanical means. This is the most common type of "Virgin" or "Extra Virgin" coconut oil sold in the market today that you will find in stores. It is mass-produced.
> 2. Wet-milling. With this method the oil is extracted from fresh coconut meat without drying first. "Coconut milk" is expressed first by pressing. The oil is then further separated from the water. Methods used to separate the oil from the water include boiling, fermentation, refrigeration, enzymes and mechanical centrifuge.[65]

Cold-Pressed – Keeping Nutrients Alive

You always want a coconut oil that has been produced using no heat, or as little heat as necessary. Generally this means "cold-pressed" coconut oil. Heat can destroy nutrients and oxidizes ingredients rapidly. Many low quality coconut oils, and this includes several that are organic, use heat in their processing because those companies can get the product out the door faster than using a healthier, slower, cold-pressing process.

Here is how one company produces their coconut oil[66]:

The fresh coconut meat is shredded (wet milled), and then cold-pressed using the water from inside the coconuts to make coconut milk. The milk is then allowed to sit for about half a day, while the oil naturally separates from the heavier water. The oil is then filtered from the curds (coconut solids). No chemical or high-heat treatment is used, and this oil contains no trans fatty acids.

So Which Coconut Oil Should You Get?

Again, as long as the coconut oil you find meets the three objectives of being organic, virgin, and cold-pressed, you'll be fine. But if you want the hands-down top quality you will get nothing but the *Gold Label Coconut Oil* from Tropical Traditions. Here is the link: tropicaltraditions.com/virgin_coconut_oil.htm

Tropical Traditions sells this highest-standard coconut oil in pint glass jars, 32-ounce glass jars, 1-gallon pails, and 5-gallon pails. The larger the quantity you order from them, the less the price per ounce will be. In the pails they come in, the coconut oil lasts a long time, as long as you store it indoors out of any direct heat.

> **Note:** Coconut oil is known as a *saturated fat.* Coconut oil is not prone to oxidation or free radical damage. An unopened jar of virgin coconut oil can last several years, even at room temperature, so feel free to stock up.

I've already told you the requirements that ensure you get top-quality coconut oil. The *Gold Label Coconut Oil* from Tropical Traditions exceeds all known factors in quality and taste. It's the best I've found after extensive searching and trial and error.

If for whatever reasons you don't want to buy Tropical Traditions coconut oil (it's expensive), I still recommend the less costly but still very good Nutiva or Nature's Way coconut oil:

amazon.com/Nutiva-Certified-Organic-Virgin-Coconut/dp/B000GAT6NG

amazon.com/Natures-Way-Organic-Virgin-Coconut/dp/B003B3OOPA/

If you have a Costco nearby, you may want to check out their Carrington Farms organic extra virgin coconut oil. I recently bought a 54-ounce jar for $15.60. By far the cheapest coconut oil, per ounce, I've ever found.

A Little About Coconut Water

A book on coconut oil really isn't complete without some mention of coconut water too. While oil and water may not mix, coconut oil and coconut water mix very well when it comes to your health and well-being.

Coconut water has been called "Nature's Sports Drink."

When most people hear "coconut oil" they really think of coconut water. They think of what most people envision thanks to Gilligan's Island and Tom Hank's *Cast Away*. Coconut water is different in taste and quality and thickness than coconut oil.

The meat of the coconut is what you think of when you see grated coconut shavings. The oil is made from that meat and not from the initial liquid known as coconut water. Surprisingly, coconut water has very little coconut taste. You may find that "boring" is the only description for the taste. Don't expect something along the lines of a *Mounds* candy bar for coconut sweetness, because coconut water can be bland.

Coconut Water Is Good

It turns out that you find some health properties in coconut water, but not nearly as many as the oil. Still, acquiring a taste is worth the effort. But it's not a massive effort because as I said, for the most part it doesn't have a lot of taste.

The primary benefits of coconut water don't even come close to coconut oil. Still, coconut water's primary benefit is as a true *hydration.* Some electrolytes are inside and a few nutrients are there for a refreshing drink. Yep, it doesn't have the taste of a traditional fruit drink, but it doesn't have the sugar either. It doesn't have the added nutrients of many "sports drinks" but it doesn't have all the unnatural stuff either.

Pure coconut water is just… pure.

Many brands of coconut water today (assuming you cannot get it fresh and assuming you don't accept anything but pure, unadulterated coconut water) can be sour. Some leave you with the same "*so-what*" after-effects that I described above. Still, Nirvana's *Real Coconut Water* uses coconuts ripened just right to give it a slightly sweet taste... and a pleasant one at that. To hydrate your cells properly, especially on hot days, have a cold *Real Coconut Water* handy.

> **Note:** Coconut waters don't have power-packed sodium that your body needs after an intensive workout. Coconut water does have as much as four bananas' worth of potassium, but intensive workouts require sodium replacement also. (You'll see in a bit what a tennis pro does to make coconut water work as an after-intensive workout drink.)

Consider coconut water to be a nice, hydrating "treat" drink that offers no sugar-laden downsides, no chemical-infused contaminants, and a heavy-duty hydrating, fresh-tasting fluid that gives you a nice change of pace over regular water.

Hydration is vital for our health. Our cells require proper hydration no matter what we're doing. While exercising, *quality* hydration is critical. Coconut water isn't going to replace most of the electrolytes you lose during intensive exercise, but it does put hydration back into your system better than plain water. So if you exercise, consider coconut water as one of several effective tools with coconut water being the hydrating tool you require.

WebMD offers a discussion of a tennis pro who swears by coconut water. See how he uses coconut water before a match to help him during the match:

> *Professional tennis player John Isner credits coconut water with keeping him on his feet for his epic 11-hour marathon Wimbledon tennis win. "It is super hydrating and has kept me going in long matches and prevented me from cramping even in the hottest and most humid conditions," Isner says.*
>
> *He drinks a mixture of coconut water and water the night before a match in difficult heat conditions and routinely mixes a cocktail of coconut water and sea salt for on-court hydration and mixes it with protein powder for post-match recovery.*[67]

His addition of sea salt (the *only* salt you should ever allow in your body) no doubt makes his coconut water mix both an effective hydrating drink as well as a post-exertion nutrient replacement.

The WebMD article went on to make this proclamation about coconut water that is worthy of attention if you exercise heavily:

> *A 2007 study shows coconut water enhanced with sodium was as good as drinking a commercial sports drink for post-exercise rehydration with better fluid tolerance. Another study reported that coconut water caused less nausea, fullness, and stomach upset and was easier to consume in large amounts during rehydration.*

Coconut Oil's Weight Loss Factors

We've already discussed how beneficial coconut oil is for you when it comes to weight loss. But some information about coconut oil didn't really fit in the 10-Hour Coffee Diet section so I want to return to its fat-fighting benefits briefly here.

Coconut oil aids weight loss. The reason is mostly due to the benefits of good fats. Fat does *not* make us fat. Quite the opposite. Unlike other good oils such as olive oil, however, coconut oil brings all sorts of additional healthy factors to our bodies that get our weight under control.

Fat and Weight

Remove fat from your diet and your body will seek a way to replace those calories and your body works harder to hang onto any fat you may have.

If you don't drink enough water, you will become bloated. Your water weight will actually increase because your body won't be as willing to eliminate fluids since you're not replacing them properly. Fat works in a similar fashion. If you reduce fat, your body does its utmost to hang onto whatever fat it currently has. Weight loss will be *improved* if you add healthy fats back to your diet.

Aisles and aisles of "fat-free" products in every grocery store in the world have done nothing but result in far fatter people. I hate to be negative, but we've sort of been sold a lie. It's time to stop harming your body and put back the lubrication it needs. Give your body more healthy fats. I know I'm harping on this. I have to. It's too important not to.

Want A More Reputable Source?

As I've said elsewhere, I am including a wide range of independent and reliable sources in an effort to verify every statement I make in this book. Dr. Joseph Mercola is another source I consider invaluable to anybody who takes health and nutrition seriously.

Dr. Mercola is someone you should know more about. Many first learned of him from his appearances on the Dr. Oz television show where he and Dr. Oz often find themselves on opposite sides of the nutrition fence.

I suggest you bookmark Dr. Mercola's website at Mercola.com. He covers a remarkable eclectic range of subjects every day and his site is an encyclopedia of videos and articles about health. There you will also find a top-heavy amount of information on coconut oil. That's because Dr. Mercola considers coconut oil to be one of the most amazing substances we can use to improve our health.

Now of course exercise is vital. Exercise helps maintain and build muscle mass, increases your dopamine (the "feel good hormone"), improves your posture and core strength, and eliminates toxins. Exercise also raises your metabolism levels and improves your ability to lose weight. But exercise isn't equal with food when it comes to weight loss. Search for the number of calories burned on a treadmill for an hour over the number of calories burned lying on the couch watching television. The difference is remarkably low considering the difference in effort required for those two activities.

Metabolism and Coconut Oil

If we want to lose weight, we need to increase our metabolism. That's the rate at which we burn calories. The more calories we can burn, the more weight we lose – all things being equal.

Exercise can raise our metabolism rate. Eating in the hour or two after exercise will burn off what you eat better than eating at other times when your metabolism rate isn't still ramped up. As you learned in the previous section, foods that raise our metabolism rate are more effective at weight loss than exercise alone.

Coconut oil is a metabolism-raiser on overdrive! As Dr. Mercola pointed out earlier, coconut oil's medium-chain triglycerides (MCTs) boost your metabolism and help your body use fat for energy, as opposed to storing it, so it can actually help you become leaner.

Why Food with Fat Tastes Better

Fat in food makes food taste better.

Coconut oil by itself doesn't have a strong "coconutty" taste. But foods cooked with coconut oil will be far tastier because the flavors are absorbed on our tongues much more effectively when fat is part of the food.

The fattier meat cuts, for example, are always considered the tastiest. And for years you've been eating the light meat chicken and discarding the dark meat and the skin, right? And hasn't that been *boring?* Just try dark meat and leave the skin on some time when you get a chance to eat a local, healthy, free-range chicken cooked to perfection. That chicken leg and skin is so amazingly better than the dry, white meat! And the dark meat with skin is healthier... no matter *what* the USDA has told you. I can change my opinion, but I can't change facts.

Often, animals that kill and eat other animals will go straight for the organs and dark meat and leave the light or white meat alone.

Don't you love hearing things like this: Put fat back into your food and the food will taste better *and* as Dr. Mercola says, "*it can actually help you become leaner*"!

Note: Look through your grocer's unhealthy products labeled "fat free" and look at how much *sugar* is added to those products! No, the ingredients won't say "sugar" but look at how many ingredients end in the suffix *–ose*. Fructose, lactose, and anything-ose are fancy and scientific terms for *sugar* when you see it on a food package. The food companies know that if they remove the fat but don't add sugar to make the product taste better, you'll never buy a second one.

Say "So-Long" to Snacking

You know as well as I that you can eat wonderful meals but snacking in between will ruin a good eating plan every time. The C's get us every time late at night: Chips, chocolate, and for some of us, cheesecake.

If snacking is your downfall, then try snacking on coconut oil! Don't get me wrong, coconut oil does not taste as good as cheesecake… and probably never will! The advantage that coconut oil gives us however is that it *reduces* our desire to snack between meals. The reason for this is that coconut oil slows down the digestion of all of our food. This enables us to feel much fuller after a meal.

Many people find that they are far less prone to snacking when they introduce coconut oil into their lifestyle.

My Recommended Dosage

If you're doing the 10-Hour Coffee Diet, stick with it. You will get plenty of coconut oil there.

But if you take a break from that or if you lose the fat you want to lose and decide to stop that diet, you should still continue putting coconut oil into your daily regimen. (I suggest you keep drinking at least one 10-Hour Coffee Diet coffee each day even if you stop following the strict plan.)

Take one tablespoon of coconut oil with each of three meals. That is not a lot, and yet it seems to do the job. That job being that we get coconut oils benefits, both its hunger pang elimination as well as the health benefits, from those three spoonful's of it. Some people advise that you take as many as six tablespoons daily but they say you should work up to that. You also might find that your digestion is smoother in the beginning if you supplement with the NOW Super Enzymes.[68]

Any time that you begin a detoxification program, when your body begins to react to the loss of toxins, the toxins are somewhat activated as they leave your body. People who detoxify after an unhealthy diet find that the detoxification itself may make them feel sick for a day or two and sluggish for a week or two.

Coconut oil does not seem to affect us so dramatically, but you might still feel some sluggishness and possible detoxification side effects – which although unpleasant is a healthy sign of good things happening – if you take too much at once on a daily basis. So if you plan to take more than three tablespoons a day, start with just three, or maybe even two for a week or so. Then add a tablespoon each week until you get to the dosage that works for you. Again, I say three tablespoons a day, consistently, will do wonders for you and you can get additional coconut oil from cooking with it.

What about Raw Coconut?

I love raw coconut shavings by the way, and they are a healthy little snack to give you a pick-me-up once in a while. A spoonful or two of coconut shavings does not spike your glycemic index the way other fruits tend to do, especially tropical fruits. In addition, you get the healthy benefits of coconut and none of the drawbacks that you get from candy, typical desserts, and fruit such as oranges that are heavily packed with fructose sugar.

Don't feel as if you need to buy an entire coconut, crack it open, and scrape the meat from the inside of the shells. Most good groceries will sell organic, raw coconut shavings and those are perfectly fine as long as you check the expiration date to make sure it's rather fresh.

Coconut Oil and Blood Sugar

One of the most important benefits of coconut oil is its effect on blood sugar. In slowing down our digestion, coconut oil helps reduce blood sugar fluctuations after we eat. This slows the rate at which carbohydrates are broken down into blood glucose, also known as blood sugar.

Coconut Oil's Fat Works Well for a Healthy Fat

The fat in coconut oil is utilized by your body to produce energy. Coconut oil's fat does not store well as a fat inside the body. It would be difficult, if not impossible, to get fat by eating too much coconut oil.

Some people do find that cheating is made worse after eating well. When someone eats healthy, such as when they eat lots of good fats, good proteins, organic produce, and eliminating most or all starchy carbs and sugars, and then they go on a binge for a week or two with lots of sugary desserts, grains, cereals, and breads, they gain an extraordinary amount of weight over what should be expected. That type of eating should always be expected to add fat to your body, but if you keep eating healthy oils, the sugar combined with the fat in the oils seems to amplify the sugars storage in your fat cells. In other words, your body knows that the oils can be used for energy so it stores all of the carbs that it can as fat.

This is my warning to you that if you go off the wagon for a few weeks, such as the month between Thanksgiving and Christmas, you can expect to gain far more weight in that month than you ordinarily would. You also will probably feel terrible as you're doing this and the food will not taste good for the first couple weeks. This is the result of your body trying to reject bad foods. Ultimately, the starchy carbs take over, and your body begins to crave them more and more, resulting in the roller coaster of increased fat weight at an ever-increasing rate.

Do yourself a favor and consider a healthy high fat, high protein, and leafy and colorful vegetable carbohydrate diet as your lifelong meal preference. Never consider this type of eating plan a short-term diet just to lose weight. By eating the way that we are talking about in this book, you will quickly feel better than you have in years and your weight will begin to shed. If you keep it up, you will find a point at which you stop losing weight and that point is when you look your best and feel great. Your body protects you in all ways if you give it a chance. People who are too thin can go on the eating plan described in this book, and they will actually gain weight until they gain enough to be healthy again. Their bodies will then stop storing the fat and convert any excess calories to energy.

This further shows that eating right is right for your body and right for you. You feel better, have a sexier body, and are in better health.

Coconut Oil and its Nutrients

Many vitamins and minerals require fat in order to be absorbed by your body. If you take nutrient supplements on an empty stomach, except for the rare ones that will include instructions to take without food, those nutrients will not be absorbed as well as they would if you had food in your body because they need fat in order to be absorbed properly into your food.

The same works for food itself. Vegetarians who eat a strict regimen of organic produce find that they do not absorb all the vitamins unless they add a quality fat to their diets. Again by quality fat, I mean a quality fat such as coconut oil, as opposed to a polyunsaturated fats such as safflower oil.

The *Journal of Agricultural and Food Chemistry* performed a study where they compared the absorption of tomato carotenoids in people who consumed coconut oil to a second group who consumed mostly safflower oil. Here are their findings:

> *"These results may have been due to the large proportion of medium chain fatty acids in coconut oil, which might have caused a shift in cholesterol flux to favor extrahepatic carotenoid tissue deposition."*[69]

These medium chain fatty acids, or MCFAs, are found in nature *most abundantly* in coconut oil. The easiest way to get adequate amount of MCFA-based oils in your body is, therefore, to consume coconut oil.

> **Note:** Even worse than safflower oil are other oils that – sadly – we use in abundance such as corn, soy (the worst of the worst in my opinion, especially for boys and men), sunflower, and canola oils. These Long Chain Fatty Acid oils contain high amounts of omega six, a fatty acid that we get far too much of.

To be clear, let me sum it up: coconut oil is a saturated fat. You have heard that polyunsaturated fats are not good for you. That is true. Those include most of the fats that are in the typical diet in the world. You may also have heard that saturated fats are bad for you too. The fact is, bad saturated fats are bad for you, but good saturated fats such as coconut oil and olive oil are not only quite good for you, they are *essential to good health.*

Muscle Mass Preservation

If you go on the typical unhealthy diet that requires you to reduce calories dramatically, you will lose pounds over time until your body rebels. When your body rebels, you will eat ferociously, craving starchy carbs especially (also known as "comfort foods"), and gain weight quickly... usually ending up weighing more than before.

Much of the weight that you lose on a calorie-restrictive diet, especially in the first few days and weeks, is muscle. Even if you exercise, and perform weight-bearing exercises, you will still lose muscle mass because the nutrients inside your body are not enough to build the muscles as you exercise. Your fatigue factor will increase if you continue to try to build or maintain muscle. There's only so much your body can do without the proper fuel.

Coconut oil has been shown to be a good preserver of muscle mass in various situations.[70]

Ketosis and Coconut Oil

Ketosis enables your body to function at a highly efficient rate so that it begins to live off your stored body fat when necessary. In other words, your body fat acts like energy that is used up instead of remaining there as storage. A high carb, high sugar diet, such as many strict vegetarian diets, keeps your body out of this ketosis state. Your body will, instead of using stored fat for energy, begin to use whatever you eat for energy. If your intake calories are much lower than the calories you consume, you will lose weight, but much of that weight will be muscle mass and water.

Coconut oil promotes *ketosis*[71] and therefore enables your body to function at a highly efficient rate, reducing sluggishness, and burning the fat stored in your fat cells for energy. As it does this, your desire for energy in food is reduced because the quality saturated fat and quality proteins that you eat to enter a state of ketosis keep your hunger pangs away. This stored body fat is known as *ketones*, hence the name ketosis.

What does this mean for us? In this state of ketosis, ketones are the preferred energy source for muscles. Ketosis helps you lose fat. Coconut oil increases your body's ability to enter into the ketosis state.

Coconut Oil Helps with the More Difficult Weight Too!

One 2009 study found that women who consumed 30 milliliters (about 2 tablespoons) of coconut oil every day, for a total of twelve weeks, not only didn't gain more weight, but actually had lowered the amount of abdominal fat, a type of fat that is difficult to lose, and that contributes to more heart problems than other stored fats on and in our bodies.[72]

Coconut Oil and Your Health

Besides weight control, coconut oil offers dramatic benefits for other health-related issues. I'll keep this simple, but I want to show you the amazing coconut oil health benefits, which can be rather astounding as more and more peer-reviewed research unfolds.

> **Note:** As I've mentioned elsewhere, throughout this book I've listed multiple peer-reviewed studies at the end of this book in the endnotes. Whenever I use a source, I tell you about it in the endnotes. You'll find that the vast majority of the sources I used for this book are from independent, peer-reviewed studies.

Detoxification with Coconut Oil

Earlier, I mentioned how coconut oil can detoxify your body. I wanted to talk just a little more about that. Every day, all around us, our bodies are bombarded with toxins. These toxins come from the air we breathe, the water we drink, and the food we eat. The further we get away from what naturally occurs in nature, the more toxins get into our bodies.

For example, living in the rural country will reduce the industrial toxins that enter the body because you avoid breathing in polluted city air. I don't believe that living in a city is unhealthy and I don't suggest that you move to the country to save your life. But it's a foregone conclusion that those in the cities will have a need to detoxify regularly more often than those who live in a rural environment.

This simply means that eating more healthy foods and exercising are even more important for those who don't live in a rural environment. By eating healthy organic produce as opposed to produce with pesticides, your body doesn't have to use up precious resources to eliminate pesticides before it works on other toxins that are in your system already.

This also holds true for municipal water systems that are generally laced with fluoride and chlorine. The next time you're at a hardware store, look at the labels for rat poison. You'll likely see fluoride as one of the ingredients. Fluoride is a killer because fluoride is *more toxic that lead.* One reason fluoride does reduce tooth decay is that it kills germs. But that fluoride, while working on your teeth, also works in your body negatively.

> **Note:** *Tom's of Maine* is a company that puts out several varieties of fluoride-free toothpaste. Make sure that you read the label before you buy because some of Tom's toothpaste products do contain fluoride. You can get the kind we enjoy on Amazon here: http://www.amazon.com/Toms-Maine-Antiplaque-Fluoride-free-Toothpaste/dp/B004M95UHI.

Anything you and your family can do regularly to eliminate toxins is almost always a good thing. You don't want toxins to build for very long and cause long-term health problems. Eating healthy and exercising are two excellent ways to improve your health because by eating healthy you reduce the amount of toxins that enter your body and you improve the fighting ability of the nutrients that you eat to rid yourself of toxins.

Getting back to our primary topic, coconut oil helps rid your body of toxins. The detoxifying effect doesn't just eliminate possible long-term problems that can result from stored toxins, but as I said earlier, by getting those toxins out of your system and your body's resources are freed up to do what it does best: running efficiently. Also, your digestive tract is better balanced and can nourish yourselves in the body more efficiently when toxins are not in the way.

Your ability to get well quicker after being sick, your healing ability after getting hurt, and your weight loss are all sped up because your body is working at peak performance when toxins are not around in large quantities to sidetrack those important resources.

Coconut Oil and Boys and Men

For the boys and men in your life, coconut oil can be more important to their health than for you. Low saturated fat diets lead to a decreased testosterone production. Testosterone is certainly affected by other factors, such as a lack of exercise and a lack of animal protein, but saturated fats are often a missing ingredient in situations where there are "low-T" levels.

The saturated fat in coconut oil is almost all oxidized for energy. The little that is not is used to stimulate and aid in the manufacturing of testosterone. Bodybuilders find that when they are trying to lose weight or lose fat for a competition, when they improperly omit all fats such as coconut oils their testosterone levels will plummet as well. When lowering carbohydrates, especially starchy carbohydrates, it becomes ultra-important *not* to limit fat intake.[73]

Candida and Other Infections

Candida is known as a yeast overgrowth in your body. Women understand yeast infections better than men probably, but an overgrowth of yeast can permeate either sex. Bad eating, especially sugars, promote candida.

Candida results in many negative effects including:

- Weight gain

- Carbohydrate cravings
- Fatigue

Eliminating candida is vital and is an important part of achieving permanent weight loss.

The *Coconut Research Center* has shown that coconut oil is effective in killing not only yeast infections, but other infections such as bacteria that causes ulcers, throat infections, urinary tract infections (a close cousin to yeast), ringworm, athlete's foot, thrush, diaper rash, and other infections.

If you ever get sick, consider taking in 6-10 tablespoons of coconut oil a day to get back on track, fast!

Coconut Oil and Hormones

I love to watch Dr. Oz. Here's something he wrote that I totally agree with:

> *Coconut oil can also positively affect our hormones for thyroid and blood sugar control. People who take coconut oil also tend to have improvements in how they handle blood sugar since coconut can help improve insulin use within the body. Coconut oil can boost thyroid function helping to increase metabolism, energy and endurance. It increases digestion and helps to absorb fat-soluble vitamins.*
>
> *Coconut oil has a saturated fat called lauric acid, a type of MCT. It has been shown that lauric acid increases the good HDL cholesterol in the blood to help improve cholesterol ratio levels. Coconut oil lowers cholesterol by promoting its conversion to pregnenolone, a molecule that is a precursor to many of the hormones our bodies need. Coconut can help restore normal thyroid function. When the thyroid does not function optimally, it can contribute to higher levels of bad cholesterol.*[74]

Dr. Oz went onto reveal even more health-related benefits of coconut oil when he said:

> *The oils found in the coconut have a positive antioxidant action in the body. This means they help our body stop the damage to other healthy fats and tissues in our body. Oxidation is considered a major contributor to cardiovascular problems and skin aging. Coconut oil can actually help our bodies reduce the need for antioxidant intake.*

Your Heart Loves Coconut Oil

As I demonstrated earlier, coconut oil is a saturated fat, but it is a good saturated fat along with olive oil and a few others. Coconut oil has no negative effect on cholesterol. Good coconut oil such as what I've described in this book tends to increase the "good" HDL cholesterol levels and improves your cholesterol profile. HDL is the cholesterol that protects your heart and that is the cholesterol that you want more of. (The bad cholesterol is known as LDL.)

> **Note:** When you get your cholesterol levels checked, the total cholesterol has very little to do with how healthy you are. What you want is a more accurate gauge of cholesterol and that only comes from the ratio of bad to good cholesterol (LDL/HDL). Given coconut oil's tendency to increase HDL, your cholesterol ratio improves, and thus, helps to decrease your risk of heart disease over time.

In the 1970s and into the 1980s when all forms of saturated fat were being blamed for major health problems in the world, incorrectly, several studies were done that showed nothing but good things for coconut oil. Those studies were the first of many that show coconut oil as a heart-healthy oil. It can actually improve the conditions for a healthy heart.

Coconut oil consumption was found to have many factors associated with a reduced risk of heart disease compared to other dietary oils namely the following:

- Improved cholesterol readings
- Lower body fat deposition
- Higher survival rate
- Reduced tendency to form blood clots
- Fewer uncontrolled free radicals in cells
- Low levels of blood and liver cholesterol

- Higher antioxidant reserves in cells
- Lower incidence of heart disease in population studies
- And more.[75]

But there's additional good news about your heart and coconut oil. The Coconut Research Center described it this way:

> *Coconut oil should be viewed as heart healthy or at least benign as far as heart disease is concerned. But there is another factor that is even more important, that reveals coconut oil as not simply a benign bystander but a very important player in the battle against heart disease. So remarkable is it that it may soon become a powerful new weapon used against heart disease.*
>
> *Heart disease is caused by atherosclerosis (hardening of the arteries), which is manifest by the formation of plaque in the arteries. According to current thought atherosclerosis initially develops as a result of injury to the inner lining of the arterial wall. The injury can be the result of a number of factors such as toxins, free radicals, viruses, or bacteria. If the cause of the injury is not removed further damage may result. As long as irritation and inflammation persist scar tissue continues to develop...*
>
> *...One area of investigation that is gaining a great deal of interest is the relationship between chronic infection and atherosclerosis. It appears that there is a cause and effect relationship associated with persistent low-grade infections and heart disease. Recent research has shown that certain microorganisms can cause or at least are involved in the development of arterial plaque, which leads to heart disease.*
>
> *A large number of studies have reported associations between heart disease and chronic bacterial and viral infections...*
>
> *...More evidence supporting the link between infection and cardiovascular disease showed up in the early 1990s when researchers found fragments of bacteria in arterial plaque....*
>
> *...You or anyone else may have a chronic low-grade infection without even realizing it. This apparently is what happens to many people who think they are healthy but suddenly drop dead from a heart attack...*
>
> *...The findings suggest that, at least in some cases, heart disease may be treated with antibiotics. Antibiotics are limited because they are only good against bacteria. Infections caused by viruses would remain unaffected. However, there is something that will destroy both the bacteria (Helicobacter pylori and Chlamydia pneumonia) and viruses (CMV) that are most commonly associated with atherosclerosis and that is MCFA or coconut oil.* **The MCFA in coconut oil are known to kill all three of the major types of atherogenic organisms.** *[Emphasis mine.-JJ] MCFA are powerful germ fighters and are known to kill dozens of disease causing organisms. Not only can coconut oil help protect you from the germs that cause ulcers, lung infections, herpes, and such, but also heart disease and stroke. If you want to avoid dying from heart disease you should be eating coconut oil!*[76]

Coconut Oil and Your Skin and Hair

Whereas just a year or two ago, you never heard about coconut oil in regards to skincare, now it seems to be all the rage. The only thing that makes me wonder about that is why didn't it happen years earlier?

An Excellent Moisturizer

The reason many commercial moisturizers seem to work, at least for a while, is because they contain a lot of water. The water makes your skin feel as though it's being moisturized well. The commercial moisturizers go on easily, feel smooth on your skin, and give you a hydrated feeling. The problem is, when the water dries your skin becomes dry again because the other ingredients are not enough to keep your face moisturized.

In addition, many commercial brands of moisturizers are said to contain petroleum-based ingredients. Just as might happen if you slathered on a bunch of petroleum jelly onto your face, many of these moisturizers suffocate your skin by closing the pores where no moisture can escape naturally.

Coconut oil on the other hand works without the tricks. And I'm talking about the type of virgin organic coconut oil that you also eat, such as that by Tropical Traditions. Coconut oil appears to help strengthen underlying tissues as well as help remove dead cells on your skin's outer layer. These dead cells can make skin feel flaky and rough.

Coconut oil puts a great shine on your hair and acts as a long-term natural moisturizer for your follicles.

Note: A little goes a long way with your hair. All you need is about a half teaspoon of coconut oil that you rub on your hair to help rid yourself of frizziness and dryness.

The Emollient Property

As you know, coconut oil contains mostly fats. This makes coconut oil one of nature's most important and powerful emollients that provide a softening and soothing effect on your whole body.

One of the reasons coconut oil works well on our skin is because its melting point is lower than our body's temperature. This means that when we rub coconut oil on our skin, it melts and this increases the levels of skin surface lipids, which soften our skin. Minor irritations such as acne and other small wounds tend to heal better when softened with coconut oil.

Itching

At this point it should be no surprise that coconut oil is not only an excellent nourishing oil for your skin, in covering your skin it soothes your skin and removes itchiness and dryness making yourself smooth and soft and gives off a glow. In the winter months, our skin tends to be much drier than at other times of the year and coconut oil enables your skin to maintain its softness and moisturized state.

Wound and Virus Attacking

Not only does coconut oil help heal wounds quicker, it also attacks viruses on your skin. Coconut oil possesses antibacterial and antiviral properties as well as antifungal properties. Not one cosmetic on the market approved by the FDA claims all of those things!

Note: Coconut oil is even being tested as an HIV virus-killing treatment.[77]

Each of these properties not only helps heal acne, but actually keep acne from occurring in the first place. The antimicrobial properties inside coconut oil kill bacteria that cause acne problems, also known as *acne vulgaris*.

Wrinkles

You already know what I'm going to say, right?

It's true. Coconut oil does have properties that soothe away skin wrinkling. It does this by attacking the free radicals that are destructive to our body and skin cells. Antioxidants are compounds that neutralize free radicals and help retard or stopped destructive reactions. Coconut oil works as an antioxidant in this manner. This means that we look younger and our skin is not only moister, but it's actually healthier. Go ahead and rub coconut oil on your wrinkles and face daily for more youthful skin.

Deodorant Usage

Coconut oil, applied after showering, has been shown to be an effective, natural deodorant in many people. For some reason, this doesn't seem to universally work for everybody, but it does seem to work for most. Just as apple cider vinegar makes an effective deodorant as well as odor remover, coconut oil seems to have that same property as well, but also appears to be even friendlier on your skin than apple cider vinegar.

Sensitivity to Coconut Oil

For some reason a few people's skin and immune systems are more sensitive to coconut oil than other peoples. This may be nothing more than a reaction to coconut oils detoxification ability. As I said earlier, when some people begin to detox through diet and other detoxifying methods such as chelation, they get sick as the toxins leave their bodies. This may be why some people's skin and immune systems do not handle coconut oil as well as others from the start.

> **Note:** Another way to get your skin used to coconut oil, if you find that you are sensitive to it, is to apply coconut oil regularly, but wash it off soon after. This enables a small amount to enter your skin and begin working while your body gets used to the effects. Gradually you can increase the amount of time between applying the coconut oil and washing it off. In general, this is a rare event and most people have absolutely no trouble using coconut oil in the ways described in this book.

If you find yourself too sensitive for coconut oil, cut down how much you use and slowly begin to increase the amount over time. Perhaps you can mix the coconut oil with some water to make it less potent when you first begin to use it on your skin if you notice sensitivity problems. Coconut oil does not have properties that tend to harm your skin. When minor irritability occurs where you apply coconut oil, this almost certainly comes from something inside your skin that is coming out and not the coconut oil itself. This is assuming of course you use a healthy, organic, virgin coconut oil.

Coconut Oil and Your Teeth

Yes, of course, I'm about to tell you how good coconut oil is for your teeth and oral health!

The use of coconut oil for healthy teeth has been known for a while. There is a process that you can go through called *oil pulling* that dramatically reduces the potential for plaque to build up that would otherwise promote decay on your teeth.

First of all, coconut oil is a powerful inhibitor of several pathogenic organisms such as viruses and bacteria. Coconut oil contains enzymes, which strongly inhibit specific mouth bacteria called *Streptococcus*. Streptococcus bacteria can lead to plaque buildup, cavities, and ultimately gum disease.

Plaque

Some people, just like animals, are more prone to plaque buildup than others. Although diet and brushing and flossing all play big roles in plaque fighting, diet and tooth care are not the sole reasons that people get reduced or added plaque over time. Even those who eat a wonderful diet, low in starchy carbs and virtually no sugar, can get plaque buildup. It depends on the person. Coconut oil can combat this plaque and do so without the health consequences of fluoride toothpaste.[78]

Oil Pulling

Oil pulling is the term applied to using coconut oil in a specific way to battle plaque on your teeth. Oil pulling can reduce plaque by 50% or more.

> **Note:** If you have heard of oil pulling before, you may have heard it used with sesame oil. Sesame oil does contribute to plaque reduction in a manner similar to coconut oil. Sesame oil, however, is relatively high in omega six fatty acids. These fatty acids you already get plenty of, actually you almost certainly get more than you should. Replacing sesame oil with coconut oil in the process of oil pulling contributes both to your overall health as well as your teeth.

Here is the process of oil pulling:

1. Rinse your mouth with coconut oil as you might with mouthwash. Work around by swishing left and right and up and down using your tongue and lungs to "squirt" the oil in as many crevices as you can in and out. It is best to do the swishing slowly while sitting down.
2. Continue working the oil around your teeth this way for 15 minutes. You can go as long as 30 or 45 minutes if you're watching television or something, but 15 minutes is certainly plenty. Doing this enables the coconut oil to "pull out" bacteria, viruses, fungi, and other debris from your mouth and between your teeth.
3. When you are finished, *do not swallow* but instead, spit the coconut oil into your sink and rinse your mouth out with water a couple of times before swallowing. This step is critical because the coconut will pull bad bacteria and other organisms from your teeth and gums and you don't

want to swallow that. (Not that we're real anxious to swallow coconut oil that we've swished around in our mouths for 15 minutes anyway!)

The best time of the day to oil pull is in the morning before you have your first meal. If you are following the 10-Hour Coffee Diet, it's fine to oil pull any time upon awakening until before your first meal even if that first meal doesn't occur until much later.

Repeat your oil pulling later in the day or in the evening before you go to bed. Your mouth will be far better detoxified as compared to brushing alone, even if you use an all-natural combination of baking soda and hydrogen peroxide to brush your teeth. Candida and Streptococcus as well as chronic inflammation throughout your body can be relieved through cleaning your teeth this way. Tooth decay affects our health in ways that may surprise you, including heart health. Dentists are trained to spot various health problems occurring in places through our bodies by looking at our teeth and gums.

Anecdotally, people who oil pull have reported rapid relief from systematic health problems including arthritis, diabetes, and even heart disease. A Naturopathic Physician named Bruce Fife said this about oil pulling:

> *"It acts much like the oil you put in your car engine. The oil picks up dirt and grime. When you drain the oil, it pulls out the dirt and grime with it, leaving the engine relatively clean. Consequently, the engine runs smoother and lasts longer. Likewise, when we expel harmful substances from our bodies our health is improved and we run smoother and last longer."*

Coconut Oil and Your Pets

I won't spend much time here, but many families consider pets to be family members also. That is why you can put small bits of coconut oil in their food every time you feed them. The oil helps to keep their coats shiny and healthy, it helps fight bacterial infections in their bodies, their teeth gain benefit from it, and they like the taste.

In spite of us thinking good coconut oil actually has a bland taste, you can put some on a spoon and your dog will quickly lick it off. In a way their attraction is just nature's normal desire to ingest healthy ingredients.

Applying Directly to Your Pet's Skin

A friend of mine once told me about her dog scratching under his chin several times a day. Looking closely she saw no redness, no irritation, no fleas, and nothing else to indicate why there was an itching problem there. So she rubbed some coconut oil under his chin.

Needless to say, it worked well. I would not be telling you about this if it didn't work. Her dog's itching ceased immediately and she did not notice it starting up again until a couple of days later where she re-applied the coconut oil and the itching stopped again. I can't tell you whether it fixed the problem for good or if there is a nagging fungus or skin irritation that still needed to be handled. If nothing else, the coconut oil relieves his symptoms of constant itching.

The Super Special 3-Day Ketogenic Coconut Oil Cleanse Diet

Writers appear to be on the opposite extremes when it comes to the word *cancer.*

It seems as though some promise that a product or a certain food or nutrient will cure cancer. On the other extreme, some writers are hesitant to say anything about cancer out of fear that they will make a promise that cannot come true. I see no reason to be at either extreme. If a certain product or food or supplement at some point has some effect, both good or bad, on our health, no matter what the area of health maybe including cancer, it is worth a mention.

You are smart enough to understand that research often shows conflicting evidence. Various independent studies can conflict with each other and often do. I am not going to make a promise that coconut oil can cure your cancer. That would be idiotic of me to do. But I wouldn't be doing my job if I were to fail to tell you about some growing evidence where coconut oil could play a role in therapy, prevention, and possible reversal of some or all forms of cancer. I will, of course, use appropriate sources.

Cancer cells can only survive from glucose and amino acid fermentation. There are ways to reduce these two activities inside your body from forming and staying long enough to cause the damage. A ketogenic cleanse has been proposed to starve cancer cells of their development and Virgin Coconut oil has been at the center of this cleanse. Its immune-boosting properties are the reason for its use.

> **Note:** Cell Biologist Otto Warburg discovered that cancer cells have altered metabolism and are not able to produce energy through normal cellular respiration. This is known as the *Warburg effect* and results in cells driving all of their energy from a process that depends upon sugar called glycolysis. When oxygen is plentiful in the cells, cancer cells lose their ability to maintain their energy.[79]

In an effort to starve cancer cells, coconut oil has been used. One of the more popular processes is called the *coconut oil cleanse* and here is the suggested way to perform such a cleanse:

1. Take two tablespoons of coconut oil every three or so hours during the day. This results in 8 to 10 tablespoons each day. (You can't eat any food.)
2. Drink about a gallon of pure water each day (meaning water without fluoride or chlorine, such as well water, or mineral water, or even distilled water) in which you can put the following: fresh lemon juice and/or organic apple cider vinegar (the Bragg's brand).

If you're of normal health, you can do this diet for one day, two days, or three days. Just note three days is ideal, although admittedly, not eating food for 3 days will be hard for a lot of people. Even doing it for one day at a time, periodically, will benefit your health, reduce your chances (or stave it off for longer) of getting cancer, and most likely give you a quick weight loss.

Dr. Thomas Seyfried expanded upon Warburg's theories and came up with this cleanse that he offers for his cancer patients. He says that fast growing metastatic cancer should go a full 10 days on the above cleansing protocol if possible.

Obviously, you will listen to your doctor and take whatever medicine procedures he suggests. I do suggest whenever you have something serious like cancer, of course, you should get a second and a third opinion. One of those opinions should be from a nonstandard practitioner, such as an acclaimed homeopathic or naturopathic physician in your area.

See if you can perform the cleanse along with the other procedures they suggest. This way you stack the odds in your favor as much as you can.

If You Don't Have Cancer But Still Want to Cleanse

For most people with a cancer diagnosis, this chapter will offer little hope because it might seem too little too late, and that may very well be the case. In addition, this cleanse may do nothing to reverse or slow your cancer. Still, it is undeniable that cancer survival rates are higher in people with lower sugar content in their bodies and it would be foolish not to at least try the natural coconut oil in this manner if you're diagnosed with that horrid disease.

For most of you, you won't have cancer. You should perform this ketogenic coconut oil cleanse for three days every few months. Doing so may not keep you from ever getting cancer, but it certainly makes it harder for your body to do so. Even more important for the short term, your body will be infused with coconut oil and its healthy effects. You will lose toxins from this cleanse and you should feel much better once it finishes. Three days is not long.

Let me rephrase what I said above in a more direct way. Even if you don't have cancer, I really think you'd be wise to do a 3-day coconut oil cleanse fast (as outlined above) every few months for optimal long term health and disease prevention! This is one of the most important tips offered in this book.

Coconutty Conclusion

There you have it!

I practice what I preach. I have coconut oil daily. I use it in my cooking, I get it in my 10-Hour Coffee

Diet coffees, and I eat and drink it by itself.

If virgin organic coconut oil is not a part of your daily routine, you are robbing your body of a valuable resource. You will not lose weight as quickly if you happen to be overweight, and you will not have the energy that you could have by adding this important and healthy fat into your daily regimen. Your health will also suffer.

16

INTRODUCTION TO APPLE CIDER VINEGAR – OLD FASHIONED HEALTH IN A BOTTLE

Apple cider vinegar – Most people fall in one of two categories when it comes to this bittersweet elixir:

1. You know all about apple cider vinegar, you use it daily for multiple purposes, and cannot imagine going a day without it.
2. Apple Cider Vinegar – ACV – barely surfaces on your radar of available products. "Something used for coloring Easter Eggs and some people use it for cooking I think."

This part of the book is for those of you in the second category. Just a few pages to go before you see its benefits and treatments, and you'll understand why it's such a necessary staple item in so many people's homes.

I have little doubt that if you read the next several pages you will add Apple cider vinegar to your daily regimen. It's not just for health. It has multiple purposes. Apple cider vinegar is one of those items that your great-grandmother knew all about, like baking soda, and lye soap that she used all the time. But today's modern world of medicines and chemical fixes somehow replaced these kinds of tried and true products.

Apple cider vinegar has been a staple item for almost 6,000 years, with evidence of its use dating back to 3,000 B.C. in Egyptian urns.

Around 400 B.C. Hippocrates recognized ACV. Yes, the same Hippocrates where modern medicine gets its Hippocratic Oath that all doctors must swear by before they can practice medicine. (They often forget the oath it seems, but that's a topic for a different book.) Hippocrates is today known as "The Father of Modern Medicine" and he strongly advocated ACV for his patients.

According to Patricia Bragg, Julius Caesar's army was required to take ACV for improved health and to keep their immune powers active during war.

I think organic apple cider vinegar will improve your chance to live longer and better.

Our Modern Health: Two Steps Forward but Decades Backwards

Today we've come a long way with modern medicine. More of us are dying from major diseases than ever before.

We've come so far in fact, that we have ignored our food supply quality and shunned powerfully active ingredients such as apple cider vinegar. ACV and other items that we find in nature are there for a reason – they work to keep us healthy. Sure, there are some ingredients in nature that harm us like arsenic.

Today, diabetes, heart disease, and cancer, along with so many other ailments were so uncommon just a few decades ago. Senility was a problem in elderly, but a minor one compared to the number of Alzheimer's patients wasting away today in shells that were once healthy and active bodies that had strong vitality.

Some people are skeptical when we say that modern advances in nutrition, science, and health have set us *back*. Surely we are healthier than ever before.

Did you know that in 1920 when Paul Dudley White invented the electrocardiograph (the precursor to the electrocardiogram, the EKG or ECG), his Harvard colleagues suggested that he abandon that invention and work on a more "profitable branch of medicine"?[80] Heart disease and related problems such as hypertension were statistically not even on the radar in enough numbers to focus on such problems back then.

A few advances in modern medicine and healthcare changed all that quickly! Now we are dying by the millions every decade from diseases that weren't even on the healthcare radar fewer than 100 years ago.

Today heart disease is the leading cause of death in the United States with diabetes and cancer following closely behind. The FDA's Food Pyramid and modern advances in heart disease, cancer, strokes, diabetes, and other troubles have done nothing to aid in the prevention of those problems.

Trillions for Cures Tossed into the Dump, Zero for Prevention

Have you considered this – In the past five or more decades, trillions and trillions of dollars have been poured into "cures" for heart disease, cancer, multiple sclerosis, muscular dystrophy, diabetes, and so many more diseases and *not one cure has been found?*

There are so many problems with that approach of constantly spending money to find a "cure."

First, it *may just be possible that there is no cure for those problems.* But even if it may be possible, is it worth decades and decades of pouring trillions and trillions of dollars into finding the "cure" when it would cost so much less to learn proven methods of *prevention*?

If heart disease was so rare less than a century ago that doctors didn't think the EKG was worth messing with, what did we do then as a people that we don't do now? The increase in problems certainly has nothing to do with medicine and medical advances because we've gone backwards. The increase in diseases *must* be related to *prevention.*

Why don't we spend hundreds of thousands of dollars to learn proven ways we can *prevent* those diseases from even appearing in the first place? Then we don't need to spend trillions and trillions of dollars to find a cure that – when are we going to admit it? – may not even exist given what we do to our bodies daily with our food sources, chemicals, deadly diets, and fluoridated, chlorinated water?

A few trillion here and a few trillion there and pretty soon you're talking about a lot of money. Could that money be put to better use? Look at the cure rate (zero) and ask yourself that question again.

Why don't researchers focus on prevention? I recently asked a former head of an Oklahoma Osteopathic Medicine Department in Tulsa how much money the American Heart Association spends on prevention as opposed to finding a cure. His answer was: "basically, nothing."

See, as long as we keep giving to organizations such as Susan G. Komen and others who spend it for "the cure" (after keeping a hefty cut), their existence and income continues. And if they ever do find a cure, they will sell the cure.

But if they ever found a way to prevent such problems, their jobs would go the way of the horse and buggy. They can't have that. So they can't work on prevention.

Paranoia? Maybe... But Pass the Apple Cider Vinegar, Please!

If all this sounds like paranoia, maybe it is. But I challenge you to challenge my logic.

I believe there was a reason all of today's major death-inducing diseases are so huge. I believe there is a reason why the medical industry consumes such a major portion of America's GDP (*Gross Domestic Product*, basically the total of all goods and services produced here)

Apple Cider Vinegar - The Cure for Everything!

In this chapter you will *not* hear me telling you that apple cider vinegar cures diabetes, heart disease, cancer, ulcers, acne, warts, obesity, heartburn, ugliness, or poverty. (I just tossed in those last two items; to hear *some* talk about ACV makes it seem possible that it could reverse even those!)

What you *will* hear me say and you'll read throughout this chapter is that ACV improves the factors in your body that make you less susceptible to problems such as most of those. In other words, ACV appears to be one of the factors that kept our great-grandparents from major problems such as heart disease, diabetes, cancer, and so on. Maybe when they were 94 and still cooking up eggs and bacon from their own farm in healthy lard they were somewhat slower than they were at 24, but they were in those kitchens living full lives and not suffering in the empty shells of Alzheimer's as sadly so many elderly folks are today. ACV and fresh-grown produce and grass-fed beef and cage-free chickens and free-range pork and raw, whole milk were their standard, daily foods. They would eat fermented foods such as pickled veggies that they made themselves, yogurt and kefir from their own healthy fresh, whole, raw milk, and they would add apple cider vinegar to their food and drink it in a glass of water when they felt an ailment coming on.

And they didn't shun desserts either! But the deadly High Fructose Corn Syrup didn't exist then and they didn't eat 22 teaspoons of sugar a day, which is the average daily consumption of Americans right now.[81] What did they have for dessert? One favorite was Vinegar Pie, and if you think that may not sound all that tasty, you need to rethink your definition of *tasty* because it'll blow you away in the Yummy Department!

In other words, the foundation of our great-grandparents' bodies was such that diseases simply couldn't get an easy foothold.

Apple cider vinegar is one of the foundations of a healthy body. Without it, you are handicapping your health. So why do that?

What Is this Apple Cider Vinegar Anyway?

Before I tell you about how to use ACV, and why you should, let's look at what it is.

Simply put, vinegar is fermented alcohol. That is alcohol that has interacted with air long enough to turn into a fermented state. Alcohol is a sugar.

> **Note:** ACV won't affect anything you do while following *The 10-Hour Coffee Diet*. For those of you on other healthy high-fat, high-protein, low-carb diets, don't let the fermented alcohol steer you away from using all the vinegar you want and need to use. The fermentation process turns the alcohol into a low-glycemic liquid, resulting in a net sugar carbohydrate value of zero. Plus, the fermentation process is extremely healthy for your gut's flora. Fermented foods such as real yogurt (homemade, using healthy, raw, whole milk if possible), kefir, sauerkraut (cold-pressed, again homemade is the most effective and it's extremely simple to make from organic cabbage), miso, and of course apple cider vinegar all provide billions – literally – of healthy probiotic bacterial units. Fix your gut and you fix all sorts of other problems and keep many problems from ever being able to appear.

It's the air that produced the alcohol to begin with. Fruits and grains such as corn exposed to the air form an alcohol. Then if the alcohol is exposed to the air too long it ferments and becomes vinegar.

Fermentation adds amino acids and enzymes to the original nutrients found in apple cider. There is no magic in the ACV itself; those active amino acids and enzymes are what do the work to make your body happy. Just as vitamins don't normally cure diseases by themselves (unless one counts scurvy that Vitamin C will reverse almost immediately), apple cider vinegar is not enough to get you well or keep you well by itself much of the time.

Still, would you want to eliminate all vitamins from your diet just because they don't directly cure you of something immediately? Certainly not. And going without apple cider vinegar in your body is another factor that can easily weaken your immune system and reduce your body's ability to fight off problems.

> **Note:** Many people on diets opt for "oil and vinegar" instead of more traditional salad dressings such as French or 1,000 Island. Dieters find that most oil by themselves on salad keeps the salad vegetables too bland. In spite of my overwhelming belief that ACV can dramatically keep your body healthier, I will say that if you use cold-pressed, extra-virgin, dark, organic olive oil on salad you will not find it to be as bland as more common olive oil. But when you add real apple cider vinegar to cold-pressed, extra-virgin, dark, organic olive oil you *really* have a taste parade in that salad bowl! It is so amazingly good that you'll never want a traditional dressing once again. (The good taste of that real oil and real vinegar combination is recognized by your body as being good for you, which results in your body sensing that it tastes much better too.)

The Acid/Alkaline Scale

Vinegar is acidic. Most people today have too high of an acidic state. We can measure how acidic we are by testing our saliva and urine's pH factor. The opposite of an acidic state is an alkaline state. In general, diseases have difficulty developing in a body that has a well-balanced pH factor or one that is slightly more alkaline than acid.

Vinegar will slightly move your pH range into more of an acidic state. In general, this is no reason to avoid vinegar except in some specific cases, which we cover a little later. The health properties of vinegar are so powerful that they more than offset a slight increase in your body's acidic state. It is the ingestion of simple carbs and unfermented sugars such as candy, corn, potatoes, and most bread (including whole wheat) that increases so many people's acidic state to such an unhealthy level and keeps them there.

Another reason the extra acid is not a traditional negative problem to your body is that ACV is good at helping you with these two health problems: heartburn and indigestion. These problems don't appear because you have too much stomach acid; they appear because you don't have enough stomach acid to handle what is in your stomach or you don't have the right mixture of stomach acid to attack the problem. ACV corrects the low-acidic nature of some stomachs, as you'll see later.

Surprisingly, good ACV is loaded with high-quality potassium. Potassium has an *alkaline* effect in that potassium stimulates the production of alkaline in your body. So although at its basic level ACV is acidic, that acid seems to know its proper role – working in the stomach – while releasing an alkaline effect afterwards by allowing our stomach walls to absorb potassium to ease our bodies back to a more alkaline state. ACV seems to be the best of both worlds when it comes to pH!

Different Kinds of Vinegar

It turns out that all vinegar is not vinegar. Not if you want the kind that aids in digestion, weight loss, and so many other things. The odds are good that if you go to the store to buy vinegar, you very likely won't get *good* vinegar. You must know what to look for. You can't go to the store, pick up a generic bottle of clear vinegar, and get the effects of pure ACV.

We will go one step further and say: the clear, generic (and name-brand) vinegars will give you *absolutely none of the effects* of ACV. As a general rule, the uglier the vinegar the better it is for you!

Although vinegar can be made from grapes, real maple syrup, potatoes, beets, melons, sorghum, rice, coconuts, and even cactus, it is the vinegar made from apples that seems to offer the most profound health effects.

Considering all the vinegars available, you may run into these vinegars:

- White vinegar – As clear as glass, often sold in plastic containers, works for cleaning, coloring Easter eggs, and does a good job at pickling some vegetables.
- Infused vinegar – A weaker tasting vinegar made from berries and herbs.
- Wine vinegar – Clear or pink in color and often sold as a wine drink in France.
- Malt vinegar – Comprised of fermented malted barley. This is the kind of vinegar you typically get to use on British-style fish and chips.
- Rice vinegar – Where is the most rice per capita consumed? Asia and that is where you find a lot of rice vinegar. Rice vinegar is sweeter than most of the other vinegars and you'll find it in a lot of salad dressings and other condiments.
- Balsamic vinegar – An Italian grape-based vinegar and is extremely expensive due to the method used to age it.
- Sherry vinegar – Traditionally made in Spain and offers a good value for cooking whereas balsamic vinegars, also wonderful in cooking, might be too costly.
- Apple cider vinegar – Made from (surprise!) apples and used in cooking. And need we say it? The very best vinegar for your health!
- Coconut water vinegar – If you buy it in an organic "raw" and "unpasteurized" form, coconut water vinegar actually comes close to ACV for helping your body stay healthy. Although ACV edges it out and is our primary focus, I'll talk a little about CWV too.

Are You Primal?

Many are now on a "primal" paleo diet, a diet based on what they perceive primitive man would have eaten. The primal diet seems to be an extremely healthy alternative to many of the fad diets out there. The primal diet also seems to be a good anti-diet, one that promotes health and long life, due to its extreme opposite food recommendations than those of the FDA's unhealthy Food Pyramid.

If you've gone primal, you no doubt wonder if consuming vinegar is legal on your eating lifestyle. Mark Sisson, one of the most acclaimed primal diet enthusiasts, recently said the following about vinegar on his MarksDailyApple.com blog and explained well how vinegar relates to the primal plan:

> "Is vinegar Primal? ... The primary component of vinegar is acetic acid, a product of fermentation by acetic acid-making bacteria. Acetic acid is a corrosive agent that can cause permanent damage to eyes, skin, and (I'd imagine) various orifices. It's even flammable. Wow. Sounds awful, right?
>
> "Not so fast. Table vinegar – the kind you put on salads – is mostly water, with around 4-8% acetic acid (which is actually a short-chain fatty acid, a la butyric acid). The dangerous corrosive agent, then, is highly diluted before it reaches your mouth. I wouldn't recommend guzzling shots of vinegar (except on a dare, perhaps), but it's not a problem in the context of normal consumption. Besides, there are actual health benefits to using acetic acid dilute, I mean vinegar:
>
> "In type 2 diabetics and people with insulin resistance, vinegar improves insulin sensitivity when taken with a high-carb meal.
>
> "Eating potatoes with a little bit of vinegar reduces the postprandial blood sugar and insulin response.
>
> "Both 15 and 30 mL (one or two tablespoons) of daily vinegar reduced body weight, waist circumference, triglycerides, and other symptoms of metabolic syndrome in obese Japanese subjects, absent any other interventions.
>
> **Verdict**: Primal. Acetic bacteria have been around longer than we have."

Which Apple Cider Vinegar to Buy

So when you go to the store and want the best vinegar, you just pick up a bottle of Apple Cider Vinegar, right? Not so fast.

Just as not all vinegars are the same, not all apple cider vinegars are the same.

Glass or Plastic?

First, if you're going to use vinegar in your food or as a supplement, don't buy it in plastic containers unless the container specifically says *BPA Free* and I've done a recent search for such containers and none seem to be labeled that. Toxins from BPA-based plastics can leech into your body sidetracking the ACV and other nutrients into handling the BPA toxins instead of working to build you up in other ways. You want glass containers for your ACV. Make sure anything else you put in your body does not come in plastic unless the plastic container clearly states *BPA Free.*

In addition to getting ACV in glass bottles, you want "raw" apple cider vinegar. Of course buy only organic or else the ACV you purchase will be putting toxins into your body that the ACV is going to have to work on before it can get to any other issue going on inside you. You also don't want any filtration used so be sure the bottle is labeled "unfiltered." This gives it a more natural look, which means it's uglier. It has brown particles floating here and there.

The Mother?

What is that yucky brown stuff floating in your apple cider vinegar?

That's called the *mother*. You love your mother, right? Great. Now you need to love ACV's mother. Anyway, the mother comes from the fermentation process and it is the live bacteria originally used to start the fermentation process. One of the ways they make healthy apple cider vinegar in large quantities is to produce some "starter" samples, which are strongly fermented apple cider batches and then grow the bacteria to produce quantities to sell. Some of the original live bacteria used to start the process end up in the resulting ACV that is sold and it is this *mother* that you see which makes ACV look dirty and yucky unlike the crystal-clear white vinegar which does nothing for your health.

If you find this brown stuff, in its healthy, raw, and unpasteurized state, in a glass bottle, you've hit the mother lode!

Bragg Organic Apple Cider Vinegar

But now that I've given you that background, can I just tell you *exactly* the brand to buy and save you a lot of looking?

You may have to go to a health food store although fortunately I've been seeing it in more traditional stores lately. Certainly stores such as Whole Foods will have it.

When you shop for apple cider vinegar, just ask where the Bragg Organic Apple Cider Vinegar is. Go to that shelf and the only decision you need to make is which size to get. Don't even *think* about another brand.

> **Note:** Bragg makes a few other products and sells them in bottles that have labels similar to Bragg Organic Apple Cider Vinegar so make sure you're getting ACV and not their olive oil or something else. If you see the Bragg Organic Olive Oil however, it certainly won't hurt to get it too! It's delicious and the healthy fat in their organic olive oil can dramatically speed weight loss if you watch your carb intake and take several teaspoons of the oil daily or on salads. Combining Bragg's olive oil with their ACV is perhaps the healthiest salad dressing possible.

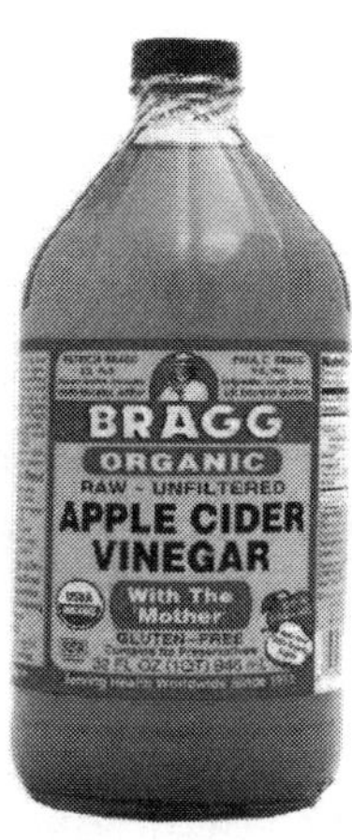

Are There Any Reasons *Not* to Use Apple Cider Vinegar?

For a very few people, apple cider vinegar may not be a good daily regimen.

If you stop doing the 10-Hour Coffee Diet and start eating too many sugars, breads, potatoes, pasta, corn, and other simple carbs and grains, you can develop an abundance of yeast called *candida*. People with bad adrenal glands do not handle these foods well and they especially do not handle the excess carbs that in a way turn into alcohol and can result in a chronic yeast infection situation. When left unchecked, candida can even produce holes in your intestinal system and allow toxins to enter your bloodstream.

As good as apple cider vinegar is, you should avoid ACV while you get your candida problem under control.

> **Note:** There seems to be a minor controversy surrounding the use of vinegar with candida patients. Some say that a yeast infection, especially a vaginal one, is treated locally using a vinegar and water solution. It is Sally Fallon and Dr. Mary G. Enig, Ph.D., who warn to limit vinegar use with candida patients in the book *Nourishing Traditions*. I don't have the answer except – in spite of how much I love ACV's benefits – I'd probably get a second opinion before using it on any form of candida/yeast problem. That second opinion would certainly be from a homeopath doctor and not a traditional AMA-certified MD. It's not that I don't trust M.D.s (or D.O.s), it's just that their pharma-sponsored training doesn't give them any knowledge in the prevention and natural remedy areas that you'll find with well-trained nutritionist, naturopath, and homeopathic physicians.

Ulcers? Avoid ACV Too

If you are diagnosed with ulcers, you should also avoid apple cider vinegar. The extra stomach acid will not help your situation and often exacerbates the problem.

Other than ulcers and yeast problems, there is probably nobody who should avoid apple cider vinegar use as a supplement for a healthy diet and lifestyle. Always let your body guide you. Your body has natural built-in mechanisms to determine whether something is good or bad for you. Many people feel better changing nothing else in their diet except adding ACV. Look for that change; it is your body's way of thanking you.

So Really, You Just Don't Like ACV?

Not everybody appreciates the taste of ACV when they first begin using it but the taste, like wine, should develop quickly and you'll begin missing it when you don't have any. Still, if you're one of the few who just can't get used to the taste, you might try what this lady did:

Nicolette from Santa Clara, CA:

"I tried ACV In hot green tea with honey and I still could not stand the taste. After reading articles online I tried vegetable juice with 2 tsp. of ACV and I could not taste the ACV at all! So if you're like me and cannot stand the taste of ACV then I suggest trying it in V8 juice!"[82]

Apple Cider Vinegar: Digestion and Nutrition

One reason apple cider vinegar helps *improve* your health instead of causing you more problems even though it's acidic was best summed up by Margaret Durst on LewRockwell.com:

> *The raw apple cider vinegar is approximately the same pH as stomach acid – so when taken, it helps digestion. [...]*
>
> *What is important about having enough acid for proper digestion is that the acid helps us digest meat and other complex foods. Stomach acid is also anti-bacterial, anti-fungal and anti-parasitic. Either having enough stomach acid or drinking apple cider vinegar before meals helps bathe our food in acid, killing parasites and bacteria that could be in improperly prepared food. This makes raw apple cider vinegar effective for preventing traveler's diarrhea and food poisoning.*

In other words, the acidic pH level is identical to that found in a healthy stomach. Improving the levels of your stomach's acid has a trickle-down effect to the rest of your body.

Digestion and Nutrients

Apple cider vinegar in your stomach means that your stomach has a better ability to digest the food you eat. Digestion isn't just there to break your big food into smaller particles. Proper digestion extracts nutrients from food and sends those nutrients through your blood into cell membranes where your body can absorb and utilize vitamins and minerals.

Whatever hinders your digestion makes you that much weaker. Whatever improves your digestion process helps makes you healthier.

Taking Your ACV

So here's what you do:

1. Pour about a tablespoon of ACV into a glass of water about a half hour before every 10-Hour Coffee Diet coffee and before every meal.
2. Drink it!

Isn't that simple?

Some of us just skip the water and drink the ACV straight to get it over with faster. This isn't necessarily easy the first few times and many can never do this. I strongly urge you to get used to the tangy taste with water before trying it straight.

> **Note:** The colder the water, it seems the less acidic apple cider vinegar feels. Colder water often equates to less puckering of the lips! So some people need to take their ACV with cold water. Warm (not hot) water actually has a stronger after-effect if you can do it. But if the puckering effect is just too much while getting used to the taste, you'll find that cold water makes newcomers to ACV happier.

Water, Water, Everywhere and Not a Drop to Drink

Don't add your apple cider vinegar to tap water! Why would you add toxins to your three times a day ACV?

A Spoonful of Sugar

It's been sang that *a spoonful of sugar helps the medicine go down* and while that may be true, I'm not too fond of sugar.

Still, as wonderful as ACV is for our bodies it can be too much to drink, either straight from a spoon or the bottle… or diluted in a glass of cold water.

One common way to make ACV go down a little easier, especially when you first begin to use it on a regular basis is to add organic, raw honey. If you buy honey at the store in bear-shaped bottles, you often are getting mud and High Fructose Corn Syrup (I'm not making this up) and both of those are not honey and they do your body no good. If you know of a local beekeeper who bottles and sells honey, that is your best source. Honey created by honeybees close to home provides an immunity effect for people in that region to protect against common allergies in that region.

If you know of no local beekeeper, you need to get honey from a health food store that sells real and organic honey.

Honey is sugar. Sugar is a toxin to your body. You should approach honey as a special treat and use it in moderation. Even a teaspoonful of honey three times daily with a tablespoon spoonful of apple cider vinegar is taxing your system with all those sugar carbs from the honey. Try to reduce the amount of honey you take with your ACV to as low of quantity as you can get by with and still be able to take your ACV.

If it means honey or no ACV at all, use the honey. Just try to reduce it down.

Note: Cinnamon helps to reduce the effect of sugar on your blood levels. A little organic cinnamon, ACV, and honey are better for you than the ACV and honey together. And it's not a bad taste combination either.

Stomach Reactions

Some people feel a slight tightness in their stomachs after taking ACV on an empty stomach, whether straight or in water. This won't be a major pain or anything, but you might be extra sensitive when you first begin using ACV regularly. Some people find they always have that sensation no matter how long they've regularly used apple cider vinegar.

If you have the same reaction, you may not be able to take ACV on an empty stomach. That's an easy problem to solve depending on how you want to approach it:

1. Take your ACV right before you eat instead of a half hour or so beforehand. Your stomach won't be quite as ready with those digestive enzymes and amino acids, but before you get too far into your meal they'll be there.
2. You might also consider taking a few almonds or sunflower or pumpkin seeds with your ACV. This keeps you from putting ACV in a completely empty stomach. Don't eat too many, maybe 6 almonds or a couple of Brazil nuts or two teaspoons of sunflower seeds. In addition to reducing the minor sting of ACV on an empty stomach, the nuts and seeds also give your body healthy fats that you require.
3. A little later I'll tell you about another way to avoid this minor stomach reaction using a combination of ACV and coconut water vinegar.

More Flora Benefits

You'll recall that fermented foods such as apple cider vinegar are good for you. They provide your stomach with needed good bacteria that helps break down food and helps you digest tougher meals such as meat.

In the early 1900s, Dr. Weston Price studied a dozen groups from all around the world who had longer lifespans than other people and who lived more disease-free than the rest of us. The only factor that *every one of the dozen groups around the world he studied had in common is they ate fermented foods!*

Some lived in ice-cold locations, some lived in desert-like heat, they were culturally diverse, some poor, some industrialized, and many of the groups lived on different continents from the others. But they all ate fermented food and they were all significantly healthier than the rest of the world.

To the extent that our cities are polluted, our environment helps to destroy production of good bacteria in our bodies. All of us can stand to add back good bacteria in our guts. These bacteria is are generally known as *probiotics*. If your doctor ever prescribes antibiotics, that medicine will help kill the good bacteria in your gut. Sometimes antibiotics are needed, but the reason diarrhea accompanies them so often is that antibiotics in ridding you of the bad bacteria don't distinguish between good and bad bacteria – antibiotics rid you of your good bacteria as well as the bad.

Supplementing with ACV and other fermented foods when you're taking antibiotics is a must, but even when you're not sick and on such medicine, the fermentation keeps your body's defenses built up stronger and if you do get sick you'll often weather the sickness more easily if you've built up your good probiotic bacteria.

ACV improves your stomach's ability to rid fungal and parasite infections because your stomach acid is strengthened with ACV. Perhaps 100 years ago and before, our lifestyles were healthier without the pollutants around us and the dangerous fluoride and chlorinated municipal water we now drink. Also, people ate healthier.

ACV will regulate your stomach. Your stomach is the entryway for all your body's possible nutrients. The healthier your stomach is, the more nutrients your body has to use.

At the Bragg Apple Cider Vinegar website (Bragg.com), an N. Roberts from California writes:

> *My husband and his whole family have lived on Zantac, Prilosec, Tums, with not much relief... just more drugs. When I heard about apple cider vinegar[...] I told my husband to try it. [...]I just started giving him the vinegar honey drink twice a day for a week. He noticed SIGNIFICANT changes in his digestion and has been able to cut back on the Tums, etc. What he didn't realize was that he was LACKING sufficient stomach acid, and the pills were reducing his acid even more!*

Always Brush Your Teeth – Just Wait a Bit!

Mom told you to brush your teeth twice a day and as usual, Mom was wise. For ACV adherents, the same teeth care holds true with one minor difference. Keep in mind that as a liquid apple cider vinegar is an acid. After you drink ACV, say in a glass of water, you should wait 30 minutes to an hour before you brush your teeth.

The acid from the cider on your teeth will do no harm, and may even help decay bacteria there. But brushing right after drinking any acidic drink, such as lemon juice, is never recommended because the acid will somewhat soften your teeth's enamel. As a general rule, don't brush your teeth within 30 minutes or so of taking ACV (or any other acidic drink).

Apple Cider Vinegar and Weight Loss

I must stress again what too many books and health food pamphlets do not stress enough: apple cider vinegar is not magic. When you get the right kind, such as Bragg Organic Apple Cider Vinegar, you get a natural food that people used for thousands of years to enhance their health and to help strengthen their ability to fight disease.

I won't tell you that the more apple cider vinegar you drink the more weight you'll lose...

... but you can *help* your weight loss – sometimes dramatically – through a diligent use of ACV.

One of the primary ways ACV helps aid weight loss is through something called *beta-carotene* that ACV provides your body with. Beta-carotene is found naturally in colorful produce and is said to be a pre-cursor to Vitamin A. Not surprisingly, carrots are called *carrots* precisely because they are rich in beta-carotene. (Or perhaps it's the beta-carotene called that because carrots have carotene...!)

Carotenes, the good stuff in beta-carotene, are fat-soluble. That means your body absorbs them far more easily and fully when you eat them with fats. This is yet another reason why getting a high-fat diet is so healthy for you. So when you eat a high-fat diet, as long as the fats are good fats such as animal fats, tropical oils, nuts, and seeds, the absorption of ACV's beta-carotene increases.

With beta-carotene's increased absorption you get more nutrients that attack and destroy something called *free radicals* in your body. Free radicals damage cells and increase your aging rate.

But forget all the science, do you know what this all means in plain English? It means you lose weight easier! When free radicals are fought and reduced, your unwanted fat breaks down far easier than before.

We Can Up the Ante

By combining olive oil with ACV on salads, as mentioned before, you're supplying your ACV with extra fat from the healthy olive oil, making your body a virtual production industry for beta-carotene and its absorption!

Say goodbye to free radicals and say hello to improved weight loss!

I Love ACV – But I Love Coconut Water Vinegar *Almost* as Much!

You might recall that I mentioned Coconut Water Vinegar and I wanted to revisit CWV for a moment. To save you time and trouble, the healthiest coconut water vinegar I've found comes from Tropical Traditions. You can order it here: tropicaltraditions.com/organic_coconut_water_vinegar.htm

With coconut water vinegar you get the similar fermentation effects as you do with ACV. Although the extreme health benefits attributed to ACV are not all attributed to coconut water vinegar, there are enough benefits to mention CWV before I move back to ACV.

Some people find that by combining coconut water vinegar and ACV they get a faster weight loss than through ACV alone. Honestly, I cannot find strict and sure references to make that claim. But I do know that a wide variety of fermentation produces the most complete stomach flora for your health.

You can stack your health advantages by making coconut water vinegar a part of your daily regimen along with apple cider vinegar to get a wide array of good bacteria. An added bonus *might* be, if reports are to be believed, that the combination of it with ACV speeds fat loss.

Better Stomach Reactions

Finally, there is one more obvious benefit that coconut water vinegar brings to those of us who believe in ACV so strongly. That is, when you combine a tablespoon of ACV with coconut water vinegar, the taste is not nearly so lip puckering as ACV alone! For the taste alone, it's worth having both on hand all the time.

I have also found through my own experimentation, that combining a tablespoon of ACV *along with* a tablespoon of coconut water vinegar in water thirty minutes before a meal completely takes away the sting that some of us get from the apple cider vinegar and water alone. In other words, some of us who have stomachs that are somewhat sensitive to taking ACV on an empty stomach do not have the same minor reaction from taking both ACV and coconut water vinegar together.

Cleansing and Detoxification

When improving your stomach's digestive enzymes and amino acid levels, your stomach's ability to get rid of unhealthy toxins such as pesticides is improved. It's true that just using apple cider vinegar, before meals as a digestive aid, *does* help your body detoxify on a regular basis.

Without toxins your body is revved up far better. It's not sidetracked trying to eliminate all the bad stuff we ingest, by desire or by accident. Your body can work on remaining strong, utilizing food nutrients, and rebuilding cells.

You've surely heard how it's important to cleanse and detoxify our bodies regularly. While it's true that detoxing is probably over-emphasized these days by the more health-conscious, increasing our use of detoxifying foods, ACV, fasting, sun exposure, and several other things we can do throughout life give our bodies a chance to do some housecleaning.

> **Note:** Sometimes it seems that no matter how careful we are at staying well, it seems that no matter what we do we still might get sick once a year or so. Drats, is it all for nothing? The answer may surprise you. Getting sick, for those who are otherwise healthy, is a *cleansing and detoxifying process that normal, healthy bodies go through periodically.* That gunk you cough up is bad stuff that your body just doesn't want hanging around. It's a good thing our bodies know the fastest way to eliminate toxins. A few days of mucus and sickness and we'll get rid of a ton of the stuff. A few days of sickness every so often is a normal process. One reason you feel so *good* when you finally start turning the corner is exactly because your body has fewer toxins to deal with. If and when you do get sick, *continue your ACV supplementation to help increase your body's detoxifying.* Plus, if you happen to have a stomach bug and don't realize it, the ACV will help attack that stomach imbalance and get you back in shape faster.

Digestion and Elimination

When your stomach flora is balanced, your digestion is better. In addition, your body's elimination of waste goes more smoothly. When you go to the bathroom you are eliminating waste products. The better your digestive system, the more waste you eliminate and the fewer nutrients you eliminate. Your body will have grabbed those nutrients from your food and absorbed them before they had a chance to be eliminated.

Regular use of ACV, therefore, improves your body's elimination indirectly. Your stomach has a better chance to do the job it was designed to do. Your kidneys don't have to work so hard to filter out the bad from the good. Your waste elimination is smoother.

Too Toxic to Detoxify

As I was writing this book, a friend of mine was about to begin chelation treatments to get rid of mercury and lead. She tested and found those heavy metals buried in her cells, sitting idle and slowly seeping until they could manifest themselves years later as something awful. By then it would be far too late to detoxify or even link those metals to the problems they eventually cause.

Note: Yes, in case you're wondering about yourself, you *should* get tested for heavy metals as soon as possible and eliminate them. If your doctor refuses to do a test *and* refuses to help you find someone who will, change doctors.

Mercury often seeps into our bodies over decades from amalgam fillings in our teeth. The American Dental Association, in spite of direct proof that mercury is toxic, refuses to make this much of a public issue because... who knows why? We suspect a bagful of lawsuits would be headed their way if they admitted that the mercury fillings (while we're on the subject of epidemic dental poisonings, we could discuss fluoride but we won't) they approved of for decades were so dangerous to us.

This friend of mine tested positive for mercury and also for lead. She has amalgam fillings so she began chelation therapy to begin removing those heavy metals from her body. The first chelation she left feeling ill. At the second one, she almost passed out during her chelation. She was also scheduled to see her dentist that week to get her amalgam fillings replaced with non-mercury fillings such as porcelain or gold fillings. But due to her problems with the first two chelation treatments, which she would need about 10 more the days following her filling replacement, her dentist told her that she was "*far too toxic to continue the chelation.*"

In other words, chelation, which detoxifies our bodies in a major way, was too hard on her body because it was too toxic to get chelation detox treatments! He said, "You must spend a few weeks doing The Apple Cider Vinegar Soak before I will replace your fillings and then you can continue with your chelation.

The doctor who said she was so toxic that she could not handle the detox treatments demanded that she start the Apple Cider Vinegar Soak that afternoon.

The Apple Cider Vinegar Soak

Your body has the ability to detoxify several ways: thru urine, feces, lungs, sinuses, hair, and skin. The skin is a large detoxification surface for the body because your skin is your body's largest organ.

To detoxify thru the skin do the following:

1. Get Braggs Apple Cider Vinegar (of course!). I suggest you get the one-gallon size, as it's less expensive than purchasing four quarts. Normally, I'd say stay away from plastic containers and use only glass. The smaller Bragg ACV comes in glass bottles. Plastic here is fine since you won't be ingesting the ACV, but using it as a soaking agent.
2. Fill your bathtub with very warm water and add 2 to 3 cups of Apple Cider Vinegar to that water.
3. Soak in that tub for approximately 45 minutes to one hour. Keep your water very warm by adding more hot water occasionally. You might want to seal the overflow drain on your tub so you can get the water deeper. Duct tape works well for that. Just don't overflow your tub.

How often you do this will depend on how toxic you are and if you are properly prepared to begin detoxification processes. A naturopathic physician can help you decide the frequency and duration.

Note: To increase your detox effectiveness, consider doing things that cause you to sweat. Sweating also helps your skin detoxify. You might want to use a sauna to achieve maximum sweating. Take some ACV in water about a half hour before going into the sauna.

Apple Cider Vinegar and Your Skin

So drinking ACV isn't the only way to utilize apple cider vinegar. It turns out that putting some on your skin can do good things also.

Balance Your Skin's pH

Your body uses your skin to eliminate all sorts of stuff from your cells. Apple cider vinegar helps to balance your skin's pH. The end result is that your skin looks better and also is softer over time.

We all like compliments! And nice skin seems to be something others recognize and appreciate.

Wash your skin with a half-cup of ACV and water. Don't wash it off if you can stand the smell. You'll notice quickly that the smell simply isn't there because ACV has a deodorizing effect, even for its own odor after touching your skin.

Bonus Use – Nice Hair!

People find that combining apple cider vinegar with coconut water vinegar makes an excellent conditioning combination for hair! We haven't tried it (yet) but the nutrients surely will produce a freshening look on your head.

Patricia Bragg, one of the Braggs who make Bragg Organic Apple Cider Vinegar, said this about using ACV for dandruff and other scalp problems:

> *The high acidity (organic malic acid) plus the powerful enzymes (the "mother's" life chemicals) in ACV kills the bottle bacillus, a germ responsible for many scalp and hair conditions. The problems caused by this are dandruff, itching scalp, thinning hair, and often baldness.*
>
> *For a healthier after-shampoo rinse for shine and body, add 1/3 cup ACV to a quart of water. Pre-mix in a handy plastic bottle and keep in the shower to use. (I suggest adding in that coconut water vinegar too.)*

Deodorant

Some people use ACV exclusively for deodorant.

The reason they do is two-fold:

1. They don't want the heavy metal toxin aluminum to seep into their bodies day after day, week after week, year after year. Aluminum is found in most deodorants. Although some "healthy" deodorants say they don't have aluminum, they do often contain alum, which is a larger molecule of aluminum. Alum is said to be far harder for your skin to absorb... but not large enough to be impossible to absorb. So staying away from both alum and aluminum seems to be best.
2. Absorption of the ACV through the lymph-like nodes under the arms is yet another avenue to get ACV into our bodies where it can do its job. Plus, ACV naturally deodorizes you. Once the initial smell of ACV drops (this takes only a few minutes; leave your shirt off until your underarms dry and the ACV odor disappears).

One final note about deodorant… if you work outdoors and find a little extra smell rising from your underarms, certainly some water and a washcloth can help take care of things. If you also add ACV to the water on your washcloth, you will find that the odor goes away faster *and stays away longer.*

Sunburns

As mentioned earlier, the sun is good for you. Enjoy the sun!

But a drawback to getting a lot of good, healthy sun exposure is sunburn. You should not use dangerous, D3-blocking sunscreens. Instead, be wise. If you're in the sun long enough to begin burning, you should cover up, wear a hat, or if you have a choice go inside.

But if you find yourself burned badly due to exposing yourself too long, apple cider vinegar gives you almost instant relief. In addition, you should have far less blistering and peeling after a couple of days. If you find that ACV stings a little, apply aloe vera oil after you cleanse your sunburn with apple cider vinegar.

Apple Cider Vinegar and Common Maladies

Although we strive to be honest and accurate in our description of apple cider vinegar and its effects, we would not be fair to ACV if we didn't address its ability to be an aid in combating some more serious problems that people have to deal with from time to time.

For example, you won't cure heart disease with ACV. ACV does, however, contain trace amounts of high quality potassium, which *does* aid in cardiovascular health and the proper rebuilding of cardio problem areas.

We're going to go through some problems that you should consider using apple cider vinegar for. You'll now always have healthy ACV on hand anyway for digestion and detoxing, why not add it to your other health regimens to boost your body's ability to get or stay healthy as much as possible?

Arthritis and Other Pains

Apple cider vinegar will not cure arthritis.

ACV does, however, help reduce the pain of arthritis. It does so by helping to eliminate waste in your cells. Toxins in cells increase general soreness and arthritis can magnify that soreness greatly. You should be better able to handle the strain from arthritis.

One forum had this to say when the topic of ACV came up:

> *My dad takes 2 tablespoons in the morning, said it completely cured his arthritis.*

Wow! Really? If this were true, that would be quite amazing. I can't guarantee that statement's assertion, but I wouldn't be surprised if it turned out to be true.

In a related benefit, bone mass seems to be helped by the nutrients found in apple cider vinegar, especially the magnesium-related nutrients. A stronger skeleton with a higher bone mass makes it easier to move in spite of arthritic pain that can arise.

Have you ever awoken to a "charley horse," a severe cramp in a leg muscle? Cramps such as those and other problems such as stiff joints are said to sometimes result from a too-low level of potassium in the body. As you know by now, ACV increases your body's potassium levels. This should help relieve stiffness and pain and may reduce or even eliminate those severe nighttime cramps.

> **Note:** Speaking of potassium, when you work outdoors a lot and get hot and exhausted, add ACV to your water. This replenishes your potassium loss through sweat as you work. At lunch, eat a light lunch but be sure and add some good, healthy, organic, raw sea salt to add back the sodium too.

Cancer

We must be clear once again. Apple cider vinegar will not cure cancer.

But one of the origins of cancer comes in the form of excess free radicals in our bodies that have been there too long. You've already seen how apple cider vinegar helps reduce your body's free radical levels. This means that the odds of you developing cancer may be reduced due to ACV and the level at which your cancer progresses, if you get cancer, may be slowed down due to the vinegar's ability to reduce free radicals in your system.

> **Note:** In an amazing study at Johns Hopkins University, vinegar helps locate and identify cervical cancer in women, possibly replacing or at least augmenting routine pap smears.

Cholesterol

According to scores of doctors and scientists not funded by agenda-based government researchers, cholesterol-rich foods do not increase your cholesterol. If you've been using margarine instead of butter, you have been hurting your health greatly. Switch back to grass-fed real butter immediately.

If you have high cholesterol, and I'm talking extremely high cholesterol, the pectin in apple cider vinegar has been found to neutralize the drastic effects of LDL cholesterol. You're helping your health every time you help yourself to another taste of ACV.

Strep Throat ACV Gargle

Carolyn from Bastrop, Texas wrote this for the Bragg Apple Cider Vinegar website:

> *"My 8 yr. old son was chronically suffering from strep throat. Twice a year every year with the last event resulting in a complete systemic infection which sent him to the hospital. It was then that I decided that reacting to strep wasn't enough, for his sake I had to find a way to keep strep from taking hold. I did my research and found that gargling with apple cider vinegar with mother would stop strep dead in its tracks. I thought it's worth a try. By chance I found Bragg Apple Cider Vinegar with Mother. When my son complains of a bad sore throat, I have him gargle once in the morning and once at night.*
>
> *Usually that's all it takes. I am a witness to the miracle of ACV with mother. It has been three years now and no one in my family that has treated a sore throat has developed strep. I can attribute this fact to nothing else except the Bragg ACV with mother. I now keep Bragg's ACV with mother in the medicine cabinet and buy it for family and friends."*

Like oil pulling with extra virgin coconut oil, I also gargle ACV as a preventative measure to ensure a healthy mouth environment.

Constipation

Little needs to be said past what I've said already. You know how good ACV is for your stomach. Constipation normally is something that will go away on its own in regular course. But an ACV user keeps his or her stomach far better balanced than those who don't take ACV on a regular basis. Your chance of overcoming or not ever getting constipated when you take ACV is great.

If you know of someone suffering from constipation who is not a regular user of ACV, consider giving them a little of your apple cider vinegar. If they use ACV a while to work on their stomachs before trying something more serious such as a laxative and the ACV works (as it very well might depending on where along the condition you entered the picture), you'll have helped them far beyond their constipation. They will be open to learning about more of ACV's benefits and you may convert your friend to an ACV believer too.

Diabetes

I just cannot stress how important your diet is if you are showing signs of diabetes at any level. Diet is extremely crucial for diabetes patients to control their insulin hormone levels and why non-diabetes people should be well aware of what takes place with insulin and health when a bad diet is adhered to.

Supplementing your healthy diet with apple cider vinegar can help reduce or ward off the effects of diabetes. The apple's pectin, still found in healthy, fermented apple cider vinegar, helps regulate blood sugar. Doing whatever you can do to regulate your blood sugar levels is always a good thing to do.

Fatigue / Chronic Fatigue

This will be easy to understand for some of you if you've studied the causes of fatigue.

Some fatigue-related issues are brought on by a build-up of lactic acid. Apple cider vinegar's amino acids can help eliminate lactic acid from your muscles, thus reducing the feelings of stress and releasing more of a relaxing state instead of a stressing state.

To help attack fatigue, especially when you need to relax the most, take three teaspoons of ACV right before you go to bed. You might combine this with a few almonds too. The fat in the almonds will increase the power of the beta-carotene in the vinegar and the fat in the almonds also helps you stay asleep.

Gallstones and Kidney Stones

It's been said that the specific acids in apple cider vinegar help to soften and even dissolve stones related to gallstones and kidney stones. According to Dr. Earl Mindell, Ph.D., gallstones and kidney stones are relatively unheard of in households where vinegar is used frequently.

Pets and ACV?

The acclaimed Earth Clinic (www.EarthClinic.com) had this to say about apple cider vinegar and pets:

> *If you have a dog that has clear, watery discharge from the eyes, a runny nose, or coughs with a liquid sound; use ACV in his or her food. One teaspoon twice a day for a 50 lb. dog will do the job.*

The web site went on to list added advantages to making ACV a part of your pet's life. Although I suspect that putting some ACV in a pet's water might ward off fleas and ticks, the following statement makes a lot of sense:

> *Fleas, flies, ticks and bacteria, external parasites, ring worm, fungus, staphylococcus, streptococcus, pneumococcus, mange, etc., are unlikely to inhabit a dog whose system is acidic inside and out. Should you ever experience any of these with your dog, bathe with a nice gentle herbal shampoo -- one that you would use on your own hair -- rinse thoroughly, and then sponge on ACV diluted with equal amounts of warm water. Allow your dog to drip dry.*

It is not necessary to use harsh chemicals for minor flea infestations. All fleas drown in soapy water and the ACV rinse makes the skin too acidic for a re-infestation. If you are worried about picking up fleas when you take your dog away from home, keep some ACV in a spray bottle, and spray your dog before you leave home, and when you get back. Obviously for major infestations, more drastic measures are necessary. ACV normalizes the pH levels of the skin and makes your dog unpalatable to even the nastiest of bacteria and you have a dog that smells like a salad. A small price to pay!

Apple Cider Vinegar Summary

There you have it. My advice is simple.

Adding apple cider vinegar to your daily routine can ramp up your health, weight loss, and overall well-being. ACV has too many uses to list and has been attributed to some amazing results.

ACV was a staple item for centuries until our modern world looked to other sources and got unhealthier in the process. Let's go back to what worked!

Apple cider vinegar is one way to easily stack a health benefit on top of other things you may do to keep yourself healthy. Do yourself a favor and make ACV part of your lifestyle.

17

JENNIFER JOLAN'S 5-MINUTE NO-BAKE DIET WEIGHT LOSS COOKIES

People are comfortable with what they do and what they eat. It's hard to get someone out of his or her comfort zone. They almost always revert back to their comfort zone regardless of how much weight they lose and how much healthier they feel.

Easy wins the health race... complicated gets left in the dust by millions who attempt it.

I want to give you the secrets and tricks that are unique and little known. Things you never heard of. *Simple solutions.*

My goal with every book I write is to WOW the reader with a lot of unique insights and tips. Well, here comes another one...

Enter My 5 Minute No-Bake Diet Weight Loss Cookies

I developed these cookies as a way to make "dieting" easier on people so they don't feel deprived of tasty and yummy foods.

Snacking, and not actual *eating*, has been a major enemy for those who want to lose weight. I've noticed through the years that people screw up their snacking more than they do their meals. These 5 Minute No-Bake Diet Weight Loss Cookies were my answer to that.

You have now heard several times that the 10-Hour Coffee Diet will help eliminate your cravings for snacks and sweets. This is true, but we all are weak at times. You probably won't need these cookies while you're doing the 10-Hour Coffee Diet since you most likely won't have any cravings (even if you did, you're not allowed to snack on the diet), but when you're off it you should consider using them.

With my cookies, I found a way to make snacking an *advantage* and not a weakness for weight loss.

An Aside: This is *Nothing* Like Dr. Siegal's Cookie Diet

I've gotten a lot of questions about Dr. Siegal's *Cookie Diet* from people who have read this. So I decided to add this quick section to set the record straight.

The information I'm about to share with you is nothing like his diet plan. And his cookies don't impress me either. Sure, it's just my opinion but it's an educated opinion. Some say that he simply wrote his *Cookie Diet* book as an advertisement to sell his branded cookies. While I have no idea if that is true or not, I've discussed his diet with several who tried it.

If a person lost weight eating his cookies and following his plan, it's because the plan has a strict limit of 1,000-1,200 calories a day. A calorie-restriction diet is a recipe not for cookies but for *failure.* Sure, you can lose weight on 1,000-1,200 calories a day. *You also lose weight on 150 calories a day... doesn't mean it's good for you.* Calorie-restrictive diets are not practical and realistic day to day and for long term weight loss success. Our bodies demand calories and they will seek them out with a passion after being restricted for a long time.

And then there's the question of Dr. Siegel's cookies.

You "have to" eat his "special" cookies. I just went to his website and checked the price of them. Hold on… sit down… get this, it'll cost a person almost $250 for 168 cookies, a 4 week supply. *LOL!* I had to laugh, sorry.

I don't know about you, but that seems ridiculous to me. And I'm being polite. I needed to get that out of the way. You needed to know this isn't that.

My cookies are nothing like his and I don't have a special cookie diet you use the cookies in. You'll make your own cookies and I've built in flexibility so you can alter the cookies so that they taste great for *you.*

What tastes good for me may not taste good for you.

I'm being practical and realistic and designed flexibility in how to make the cookies. Feel free to make slight changes to get the taste right so that you can enjoy having these cookies for a long time.

As you'll see a little later, these cookies will cost you no more than 15-20 cents each, or about $1 a day. That is a bargain if you've priced even traditional store-bought cookies lately. But – to be clear since I know you're probably doing mental arithmetic, no, that's not $30 a month in addition to what you already spend on food. Not at all. First, you can do what you want with this information.

You don't need to follow my suggestions on how many and often to eat the cookies each day. You can also skip days. You can modify them depending on your current goals.

You are entirely in charge of when and how often you have the cookies.

Second, if you were to follow my suggestions on how many cookies to eat and how often to eat the cookies, please remember that the money spent on the ingredients for the cookies would be offset by less money spent on other snacks and foods. Most likely, you can expect to *save money* since most people spend more than $30 a month on snacks.

Let me summarize: I don't make any money if you decide to create and eat the weight loss cookies I talk about here, unlike Dr. Siegal, who does make money on his own cookies. (And it's a *lot* of money, $250 for a month's supply of his cookies. Crazy isn't it?)

The 5-Minute No-Bake Diet Weight Loss Cookie Recipe

The cookie ingredients are listed below:

- 1 to 1.5 cups of old-fashioned oatmeal (raw oatmeal, don't cook it… and *no,* don't use instant oatmeal). It is best if you get organic *oat groats* and roll them yourself with a small hand mill into oatmeal flakes. You get the most nutrients this way. However, this is not necessary.

- 2 to 3 scoops (40 to 75 grams of protein) of your favorite protein powder (doesn't matter which flavor you choose). Use a good whey protein. Don't use a soy protein powder.
- 4 tablespoons of Almond butter
- 1/4 cup of either whole milk or filtered water. Raw, whole milk is best and the healthiest. You can also use Almond or Rice Milk if you want, but of the two I strongly suggest almond milk.

Mix it all up in a bowl. That's it.

Four ingredients. In the above amounts that I listed, you will be able to ball up about 6 to 7 cookies.

You are free to adjust the amount of each ingredient. Play around with it and find what you like. I'm not an expert at baking things. In fact, I'm pretty bad in my opinion.

Note: The cookies will be a bit "soupy" when you make them, so you should put them on a baker's sheet/pan and put them in the fridge for an hour to allow them to solidify.

Expect your hands to get really messy when making these cookies.

In addition to the 4 ingredients for the basic cookies, here are some other ones that you can creatively add in to the mix to improve or change the taste or to make them healthier:

- Wheat germ
- Cinnamon
- Chocolate chips
- Coconut flakes
- Squeezed juice from 1/2 of a lemon
- Vanilla extract or other extracts
- Milled flax seed
- Cacao powder

Feel free to add any of these ingredients to the mix when making the cookies. Experiment and find what you and your family like.

The primary reason why these are great cookies to snack on while on a diet has to do with the fact that they're high in protein and healthy fats. Most snacks are processed garbage. Other "healthy" snacks aren't as healthy as we've been told.

Replacing those snacks with protein cookies will help your weight loss cause. You're replacing bad calories with healthier (and more filling) calories. Besides, everyone loves to eat cookies!

So, how often and how many cookies should you eat?

That's up to you and what type of diet you're currently on. If you're not on any specific diet, just use these cookies as your primary snacks. Eat one to two cookies each time you snack on them.

Costs

Here's a breakdown of the cookie costs:

- Old fashioned rolled oats (18-ounce container) = $1.50. The cost per batch of 7 cookies is about 15 cents.
- Protein powder: Prices vary depending on brand, size of the container, etc. Figure on a cost of around 75 to 80 cents for each batch of 7 cookies.
- Almond butter is about $4 for a 12-ounce jar (from Walmart). This comes out to about $1 for each batch of 7 cookies.
- Milk and water... water is obviously free and milk would average out to about 20 cents for a batch of 7 cookies

As you can see, the costs are quite reasonable and not too expensive when you compare them to the costs of the snacks you're currently having.

Frequently Asked Questions

Q: Can I put them in the oven for 5 minutes to dry the cookies out?

A: Yes you can, if you want. But it's not necessary. You can also put them in the fridge for about an hour to solidify the cookies.

Q: How fast will I lose weight?

A: The cookies alone are just one part of a weight loss strategy. I have no idea on many other aspects such as your overall diet, your exercise program, whether or not your hormones or brain neurotransmitters are out of balance and need fixing, how well you sleep, if you're taking any type of medications, your stress levels, or many other important aspects that play a role in weight loss.

To answer how fast you will lose weight eating these cookies… there really isn't a way I can answer that since there are so many other factors that affect weight loss.

Why do these cookies help with weight loss? The short answer is that weight loss begins through the use of protein from the protein powder and the good fats from the almond butter.

But also, you are switching in good calories and switching out bad calories. You're blocking out bad calories by eating these filling cookies. If you additionally sprinkle in some cinnamon, you'll also get a nice insulin sensitivity boost.

Another benefit of these cookies is they destroy hunger cravings due to their high protein and fat content. This will help you to avoid calorie-dense, processed garbage snacks.

Q: Can I eat these cookies with meals?

A: Yes! These cookies make a great addition to your meals. The added protein and fats help to slow down the digestion of the carbs from the meal.

Note: Eat these with your actual 10-Hour Coffee Diet meals and *not* with the 2 to 3 coffees.

If you're going to eat these cookies with a meal, I suggest you eat one or two of them a few minutes before the meal.

The reason behind that is to help "pre-fill" you up. The more unhealthy the meal you're going to eat, the more you should consider eating one or two of these cookies before it. This way you'll end up eating less of the meal. This is a calorie-blocking strategy.

Pictures

Here are some pictures from the cookie-making process. The first picture is of the ingredients. The second picture is of the ingredients unmixed in the bowl. The third picture is of the ingredients mixed up in the bowl. The fourth picture is of the cookies.

Note: You don't need to use all of the ingredients shown in the ingredients photo.

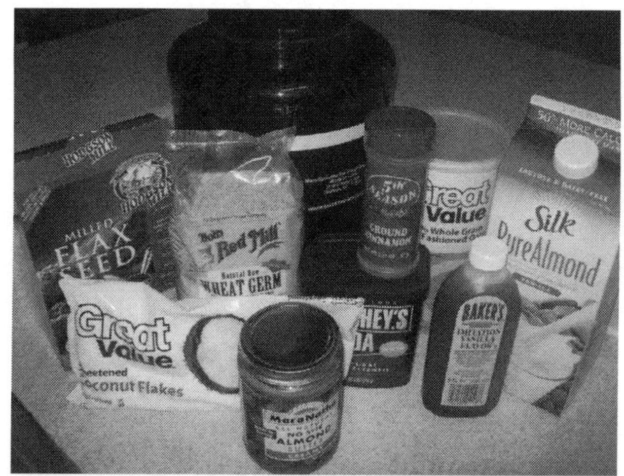
MILLED
FLAX
SEED
Bob's Red Mill
WHEAT GERM
Great Value
Great Value
Silk
BAKER'S
ALMOND

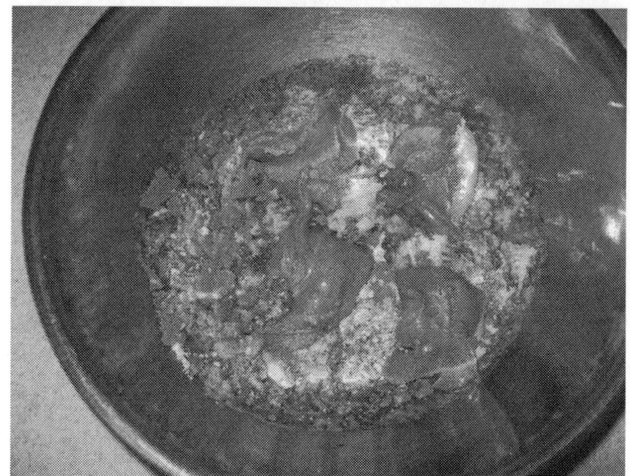

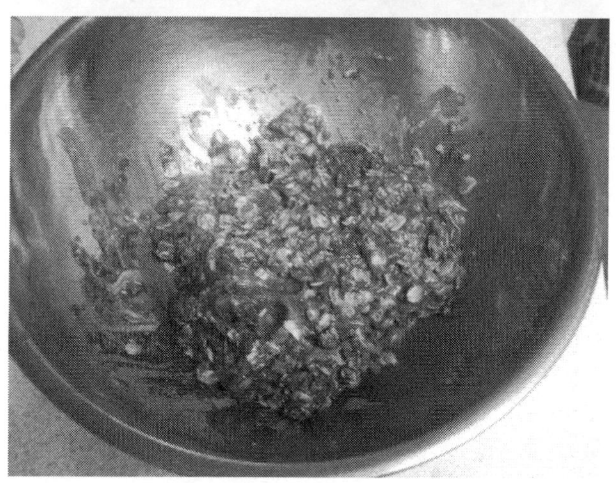

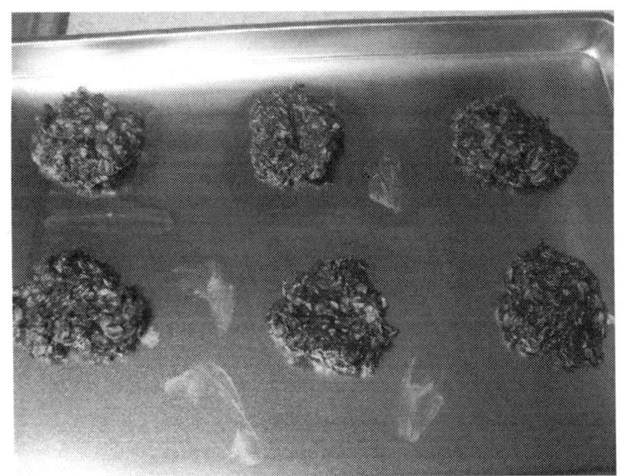

18

15-SECOND DIET TRICKS: TURN BAD MEALS INTO "WEIGHT LOSS" MEALS INSTANTLY!

This chapter begins your small journey into 15-second diet tricks, an amazing weight-loss concept that has proven popular. Absolutely nothing here departs from or takes away from the 10-Hour Coffee Diet. You can enhance virtually any diet plan with the 15-Second diet tricks.

The 15-second diet tricks consist of nothing more than two tips. But these two tips are *powerful.* And even better, they are as easy as they are powerful. And it's my guess that you've never heard of these two tips before. But they will change the way you view diets.

My bottom line goal is this: I'm going to show you how to turn bad meals into good meals and good meals into great meals.

If you're looking for something simple and quick to do to help you along in losing weight or maintaining your weight, these two tips are perfect for you. And the greatest thing about these two tips is that they don't involve you going on a diet or changing how you eat. You can relax.

Obviously, the healthier you eat combined with eating in moderation and doing plenty of exercise, the more likely it is that you'll lose more weight.

I'm going to be realistic and assume most people hate diet restrictions and aren't particularly consistent with their exercising. We know people hate diet restrictions and long, boring exercise routines because so many people who begin them never continue with them. Keeping you on the right path is where these two tips come in.

Your Weight Loss

If you're gaining weight and need a quick fix to help stop more pounds from piling onto your body, definitely give this a try. I can't guarantee that you'll lose weight because I don't know you and I don't know how you'll use the following information. As with anything, the more serious and diligent you are, the better the results will be.

While these tips work for most people who have used them, there will always be people that these tips don't work for. This can occur for a variety of reasons. But most often it's usually the result of a half-hearted attempt.

What I can promise you is that these two tips most certainly will help you to maintain and possibly lose weight while improving your health if you give them an honest try for just one month. That's all I ask.

Each of the tips takes only 15 seconds to do. In other words, the time it takes you to read this short paragraph is about as long as these two tips take! Given how short they are, hopefully they'll develop into healthy daily habits that you do all the time for the rest of your life.

These two tips offer a complete benefit package for you. They not only help your weight and can improve how your body looks, but more importantly these two tips are great for your health. With health care costing skyrocketing these days, every little bit of preventative maintenance work on your health will add up to saving you thousands of dollars in future health care costs.

15-Second Diet Trick #1

Modern diets have lost sight of what makes food taste good. Spices make food taste good. Plus, many spices are good for us. You might faintly recall sitting in high school history class learning about spice trade routes and spice wars. The reason countries went to war over spices is precisely why we should take a new look at these ancient additives. Spices taste good and are good for us.

The first of the two 15-Second Diet Trick tips here uses one of the most loved spices in use today. The tip is simple:

> *Sprinkle cinnamon on whatever it is you're eating. Yes, this includes your 10-Hour Coffee Diet coffee! (Cinnamon doesn't always mix well and often just floats on top of your drinks. This means for your 10-Hour Coffee Diet coffee, add cinnamon in the blender before you blend the drink. But even for drinks you don't blend, cinnamon tastes good stirred into coffee, tea, and even milk.)*

If you don't want to sprinkle cinnamon on your food, just sprinkle cinnamon into whatever it is you're drinking with your meal and take it that way.

Some people actually sprinkle a little cinnamon directly into their mouths and then quickly take sips of a drink to wash it down. It's up to you how you take cinnamon, but just be sure to take some cinnamon whenever you eat something.

Cinnamon has a blocking effect when you eat something extremely bad such as a fattening, sugary dessert. When you eat something bad like that, something with a lot of sugar and carbohydrates in it, cinnamon is extremely important. Cinnamon slows down the effects of carbohydrates on your body.

And one of the best things about cinnamon... cinnamon is cheap. I sometimes get the little spice bottle of ground cinnamon from Walmart. It's under a dollar and contains 2.37 ounces (67 grams) of ground cinnamon. See, I told you it was cheap… but you probably already knew that. If you're not in the USA or don't shop at Walmart, I'm sure you could easily find some cheap ground cinnamon at your local grocery store in the spice aisle.

The little spice bottle of ground cinnamon usually lasts about 4-7 weeks for most people who sprinkle a little bit of it on their food 2-3 times a day. The total cost to you for using this weight loss trick is under one dollar for a month or so.

Note: You can stack the advantages of cinnamon if you buy organic cinnamon. You pay more for organic over conventional but your body has to consume fewer resources to throw off any toxins that conventional cinnamon may contain.

These three kinds of cinnamon are most common:

- Saigon
- Ceylon
- Cassia

Cassia is the most common. If the cinnamon you buy isn't marked, you'll probably get Cassia. Cassia is in the middle in how effective it is at reducing the effects of carbs on your body. Saigon has the best effect of the three in reducing any carb impact so if you don't mind paying a little more, Saigon will be more beneficial over cinnamon that isn't marked. Ceylon has the least impact on reducing carb damage to your body, *but* Ceylon has one huge advantage: In quantities of more than a teaspoon and a half a day it is not toxic. Saigon and Cassia in quantities of more than a teaspoon and a half daily *can* be toxic.[83]

How much should you sprinkle on your food or how much should you take with a meal? Research suggests that about a half teaspoon each time will give you full impact. Although I don't measure how much I use, I use somewhere around a half teaspoon on my food each time I use it.

Now you're probably thinking that it'll be weird to put cinnamon on all the different types of foods you eat. Or that it may taste weird. The truth is, yeah it is kind of weird. But it's worth it. As far as taste goes, after a few days or at most a week, most people barely even taste the cinnamon because they've become so used to it. I love the stuff so it never has a negative effect on foods I eat.

Now, do you need to put the cinnamon in or on all meals? Ideally yes. Realistically, that won't be possible. If you're on the go, you can bring the little cinnamon bottle with you. It's small. But then maybe you don't want people to see you sprinkling cinnamon on your food because you don't want them to think you're weird.

That's understandable and in some situations even I don't use cinnamon on my meals, but for the most part, don't worry about it. This is your health and your body. Nobody cares. Your waiter or waitress doesn't care. (I do get questions when they see my empty iced tea glass that looks like a bunch of mud has been mixed in with my tea!)

In fact, sprinkling cinnamon on your food will lead to some interesting conversations with people. Just tell them it's a cool weight loss trick you learned that manipulates insulin sensitivity… and that it only costs less than a dollar a month to do.

Bonus Benefit for Children

There's one major cinnamon advantage you should know about before I get into the "why" explanation. If you have children, one of the best things you can do for their health and to help them avoid type-2 diabetes that's become so prevalent in the Western World is to sprinkle cinnamon on their food.

This is totally safe for children; just make sure they get less than a teaspoon and a half a day if it's not Ceylon. I do this for my kids. This gives them a huge "health advantage" over other kids as they grow up.

In fact, as powerful as cinnamon is for the health and weight of adults, it's even more powerful at preventing growing kids from getting fat.

Remember, cinnamon is a natural spice. Don't fear it. It's not a drug.

Use your foods as medicine. It's not only cheaper than prescription and over-the-counter drugs, it's healthier… and it's *natural.*

Why This is So Critical

I want to address why cinnamon is so great for weight loss and health.

First off, cinnamon increases your sensitivity towards insulin and decreases your blood sugar levels. There is a kind of interplay always going on between insulin and blood sugar. When you eat and swallow food, your body turns that food into glucose. Glucose is the main source of energy for your muscles and brain.[84]

Now, if you eat a lot of ice cream or a bunch of fries that have a lot of sugar in them, such sugars move into your blood stream quickly, unlike proteins and fats. What then happens is your body gets a serious amount of blood sugar flowing. This blood sugar forces your pancreas to dump a lot of insulin in order to fight off the spiking of your blood sugar levels.

It is your insulin's job to regulate sugar metabolism and shuttle the blood sugars (glucose) into your cells where it's later used for energy. In simple terms, it's like a tug-of-war between insulin and your blood sugar. The blood sugars (glucose) want to stay in your bloodstream while insulin wants to get them out of the bloodstream and into the cells.

And in this tug-of-war, your body is waiting to see which side wins to see what it has to do. And it will always do one of two things: gain weight or lose weight. If blood sugar levels are too low, that signals your brain that you're hungry and need calories even if you just ate a half-gallon of ice cream.

This is the reason why people often get hungry soon after eating.

The problem is that when you eat in a manner that requires your body to release a lot of insulin often, you eventually become *insulin resistant.* That means the insulin doesn't have the same effect on you as it should... and as it used to. You in fact need more amounts of insulin to get the job done in fighting high blood sugar levels.

In other words, your body starts over-producing insulin.

This over-production of insulin and insulin resistance leads to type-2 diabetes. When you have type-2 diabetes, your liver and muscle cells don't normally respond to insulin. This results in the blood sugars (glucose) not getting into the cells to be stored for energy.

When the blood sugars get blocked out of your cells and liver, it results in really high levels of blood sugars building up in your blood. This causes *hyperglycemia.* When this occurs, the insulin your body produces simply can't keep up with your body's demands. This results in symptoms such as you being tired, hungrier, and thirsty *more often.*

Now, suppose you begin sprinkling good old cinnamon on everything. Cinnamon has a compound called MHCP. This insulin-mimicking compound essentially sensitizes and activates the receptors in cells for insulin. Thus, with cinnamon you become sensitive to insulin (insulin sensitive) instead of becoming resistant to insulin (insulin resistant).

Basically, you can avoid all that bad health stuff mentioned above. Cinnamon has the ability to correct your body's reaction to sugar. And that's a great benefit.

Taking cinnamon (especially with a bad meal that's high in sugars) will do a lot towards harmonizing insulin and blood sugar in your body. Instead of being at war, your insulin and blood sugar are at peace and work with each other.

Note: If you do sprinkle cinnamon directly into your mouth, be aware that for some people, it will irritate the tissues in your mouth. Do it that way as a last option.

Anyway, it takes less than 15 seconds to sprinkle cinnamon on your food and the effects on your health and its ability to help you lose weight is well worth it. And it'll last over a month while costing less than a dollar!

Just to emphasize this because I don't want you to take this information lightly, ground cinnamon is *almost magical* with its health benefits.

You don't want to chance having type-2 diabetes if you can avoid it. The scary thing is most people who have type-2 diabetes don't even know it. What's even scarier… while not *everyone* with type-2 diabetes is overweight, obesity and lack of activity are two of the biggest causes of this type of diabetes.

The bottom line?

Use cinnamon to turn a bad meal into a good meal... or at least a lot better meal. You'll save your health, which will save you a lot of money, and you'll also improve your body in the process. When you use cinnamon and then add the next 15-second diet trick into the mix, your body *really* responds!

15-Second Diet Trick #2

The second 15-second diet trick is even more powerful than the first. And just as easy! Enter leucine and BCAA's.

The Food We Eat is Food We Shouldn't

As you probably know by now, most foods we eat these days is low quality food. The food is processed to death, it comes packaged, and it's essentially dead nutritionally.

If that's not enough, people further kill the nutrition in their food by putting it in the microwave. There's a reason why there's the saying "nuke it." Your microwave is taking up precious counter space in your kitchen. Throw it out so you're not temped to use it *ever* again. Your kitchen should be the place where you prepare healthy, good-tasting meals for you and your family and not the place where you destroy food.

Today's "good" foods, such as fruits and vegetables, are low quality compared to the fruits and vegetables people ate fifty or more years ago. This has to do with all the pesticides and herbicides sprayed onto them to keep the bugs and pests from eating them up or destroying them, the poor soil quality they grow in, the distances they have to travel before getting to your table, and the fact that most fruits and vegetables these days are genetically-modified (GMO).

All in all, such food not only tasted better years ago, they were packed with nutrition.

To put it bluntly, our society has come a long way technologically, but when it comes to food we buy crappy food and we have bad food habits. We need all the help we can get when eating. We can't go without eating, although the 10-Hour Coffee Diet coffees help on that issue.

Solution to Food Pollution

I harp about organic produce a lot. We are all on a budget. And we must strive to eat as healthy as possible, but sometimes it's true that our budgets just don't always let us eat as pure of food as we want. Plus, when we eat out or over at a friend's house we usually have little or no control over the food served. And our kids love to eat at Chik-fil-A and other fast food places and you know how it is... sometimes such garbage food, in spite of our best intentions, efforts, and knowledge... Just. Sounds. Good.

So we need a boost to help our bodies. We don't live in food laboratories where every ounce of our food and drinks are perfect. We want to enjoy life. Those of us who strive to eat as healthy as possible enjoy life more than those who don't – I'm convinced of that. But we also eat a lot of bad with the good just because that's life today.

We need help to turn bad foods into a good meal. That's where *leucine powder* and *branch chain amino acids* (*BCAA*'s) enter the picture.

Comparing the Two

Here's a quick rundown of BCAA's and leucine and what they can do for you.

BCAA's are the building blocks of your body. Proteins are made up of amino acids. These proteins comprise about 35% of your muscle mass. They need to be present for molecular growth and development to happen.[85] This is all vital because the job that BCAA's do include all this:

- Cell building
- Tissue repair
- Antibody development
- Enzyme and hormone production
- Improved oxygen movement throughout your body.

Leucine is the most important part of BCAA's.

A Short Detour into Why We Get Fatter as we Age

We could take the science much deeper, but really the most important and relevant thing to understand is this: as we age, we naturally lose muscle mass at a faster rate. If you do nothing, you'll lose 5% of your muscle mass every 10 years starting at the age of 35.

If you're a woman, I understand that you may not want bulky muscles. Bulky muscles are not an issue here, though. You do *not* want to lose the muscle mass that you have. When you lose muscle, you automatically slow down your metabolism. When metabolism becomes slower you lose fat slower.

Why? This occurs because muscles are more metabolically active than fat. Each pound of muscle burns up to ten more calories a day compared to each pound of fat. This occurs *even when you sit around doing nothing!* The amount of energy (calories) you burn at rest is your basal metabolic rate (BMR). The release of energy (burning of calories) in your BMR state is only for basic survival.

Consider this: if you lost one pound of muscle a year, you'd lose the ability to burn off 3,650 calories (365 days x 10 calories) or one pound of fat. This means that if you lost a pound of muscle, you'd end up gaining a pound of fat in one year, all things being equal. Sadly, your scale weight may be the same, but your body won't look as good.

The older you get, the more muscle you naturally lose. So basically, without doing anything, you'll gain at least one pound of fat a year after the age of 35. That's the bottom line and sadly it goes straight to our bottoms and waistlines.

Obviously, the better we eat and the more effectively we work out, along with balancing your brain chemicals, the more we fight the battle between aging and muscle loss. In eating and exercising wisely we can gain some new muscle.

Here's the critical thing for *everyone* reading this: Even if you're younger than 35, this still applies to you! Muscle loss is only more pronounced the older you get. But younger people lose muscle also, just at a slower rate. I emphasize age here only because the rate increases with age, but it happens to all of us. It still happens with young people if they don't treat their body right.

More About this Special Diet Trick

Because you cannot constantly eat "healthy" foods, your body is surely struggling to maintain its muscle mass. As sad as this may sound, our bodies don't consider muscle mass essential to survival. Therefore, it will try to shed the extra weight whenever possible to make "survival" easier.

Maintaining muscles requires *more calories*. But our bodies try to do the most with the least and knowing that more calories requires effort, our bodies will shed muscle before fat.

As you may have guessed by now, leucine and BCAA's help preserve your muscle mass. They do this *even if you eat bad foods and even if you are literally starving.*

But there is a catch. The key to their effectiveness is timing and dosing. You need to time when you use either of them and you need the proper dosage. Take this seriously, be strict about the timing and dosage details I'm about the give you.

To get the most out of leucine powder or BCAA's, take them right before meals and right before you workout (if you workout). The reason you need to take leucine powder or BCAA's before you eat is because they help unleash the full potential of your food by as much as 70%. That's what I mean when I say these almost magic supplements can turn a bad meal into a good meal.

Let me make an extreme example: I don't recommend it, but if took leucine before you eat three bowls of ice cream, you'll basically wipe out most of the "badness" of the ice cream because leucine and BCAA's are so good for you.

Note: Always stack your advantages! Remember cinnamon's benefits! To further reduce the ice cream's damage, you would sprinkle cinnamon on the ice cream too.

Bonus: Although I'm using ice cream as the example, taking leucine with a meal that contains some protein works *even better.* This is because it acts as a sort of "boss," or catalyst, to other proteins and amino acids and enables your body to utilize them more efficiently.

The Dosage

I recommend you use five grams of leucine powder over five grams of BCAA pills. You should see a slightly more dramatic effect. But there's a trade-off: Honestly, leucine powder tastes horrible.

You can help this however. I take a small five-gram scoop of leucine powder, throw it in my mouth, and then drink something as fast as humanly possible to wash it down my mouth. This takes less than 15 seconds to do. If that's too caveman for you, add it to a protein shake or a green smoothie. Of course, leucine powder needs to be in your system right *before* you eat so it's best to find a way to get it into you without mixing it with food such as a smoothie.

Of course, you can mix it into your 10-Hour Coffee Diet coffee. That helps mask the flavor and "powers up" the coffee even more.

There are two reasons why I recommend leucine over BCAA's even though you have to work around the bad taste:

1. Research has shown that leucine is *by far* the most important of the branch chain amino acids (BCAA's) for muscle protein synthesis. In other words, no matter how much or little protein or amino acids (other than leucine) you take, the muscle protein synthesis is entirely controlled by how much leucine you have in your bloodstream. So the other BCAA's are kind of pointless, to a degree.
2. Leucine powder is cheaper than BCAA pills.

If you're in the USA or Canada, here is a link to the leucine powder I personally buy: amazon.com/Serious-Nutrition-Solutions-Leucine-Grams/dp/B004K5ZYIY/.

500 grams for under $35 (at the time of this writing) is a steal considering its power. Although it may not be *extremely* cheap like cinnamon, it's also not *too* expensive.

If you took two five-gram scoops a day, your leucine would last 50 days. I prefer you take three five-gram scoops a day, once before (or at the start of) each of three meals (say two of your 10-Hour Coffee Diet coffees and one meal) and that'll last you 33 days.

Remember to take it before each workout. (You can switch out taking it from one of the meals or coffees if necessary.) Doing so improves you recovery, reduces muscle breakdown, and helps to preserve or build muscle.

Yes, you can use BCAA's. I prefer you don't, but since leucine is hard to find in pill form, I realize some people are extremely picky and won't want to put bad tasting leucine powder in their mouths. They simply won't do it regardless of the benefits and even though the bad taste in the mouth only lasts a few seconds.

So my second, slightly less effective, and definitely more expensive option is to use BCAA pills instead. That negates the taste problem. BCAA's have leucine in them, but they also have 2 lesser amino acids in them as well. Since we established that leucine is the king of amino acids, we want to use as much of that as possible. By taking BCAA's, you're diluting out some of the leucine.

But whatever you do, do something! Leucine or BCAA's, both ways you're leap years ahead of those who don't take either. If you're in the USA or Canada, here's a BCAA I recommend (although you can find them at your local health food store, Amazon, or GNC): bodybuilding.com/store/opt/bc.html

400 capsules cost $24. Since every two capsules contain just one gram of BCAA's in them, you'll need to take ten capsules before each meal or before working out. Yep, it's a pain compared to taking leucine powder. Plus, since there's less leucine in the pills, it's not as effective.

But those BCAA pills are still extremely effective compared to nothing!

Note: Taking ten capsules, three times a day is obviously 30 capsules a day. So the 400 capsule bottle would last you about two weeks. As you can see, it's more expensive than the leucine powder.

In Summary

In reading this chapter, you have learned more about the mechanisms and nutrients behind muscle mass and fat storage. Still, everything I wrote above can be boiled down into extremely simple tactics:

1. Take a half-teaspoon of cinnamon with each meal (no more than one and a half teaspoons daily).
2. Take five grams of leucine powder *or* five grams of BCAA pills before your meals and before working out, a total of 3 times a day.

By using these two powerful diet tricks that take just 15 seconds each, you'll immediately begin of turning bad meals into good meals.

19

COSMETICS CAN HELP US LOOK GOOD BUT FEEL BAD

I often hesitate to believe initial reports I hear from health-related websites when it comes to extreme benefits or extreme problems associated with any product. For example, you already know how much I love apple cider vinegar, not for its taste, but for its fermented health-producing qualities as well as all it can do for skin, hair, and help in other ways.

I spent several pages warning you that apple cider vinegar does not cure cancer, cure baldness, or make you richer. It seems as though promise after promise is made about apple cider vinegar, as well as other quality products, that simply don't hold up to scrutiny.

I think overpromising hurts the cause. The same goes for making crazy warnings.

It turns out that it's actually difficult to overstate some of the dangers that many cosmetics have caused over the years to the public health. Sadly, the list includes maladies like these:

- Liver damage
- Kidney damage
- Neurological problems
- Skin diseases
- Cancer
- As well as others

Like Food, Cosmetics Can Be Unnatural

Many cosmetics are just a mishmash of lots of chemicals, many of which have a short-term positive effect on our skin, but have a long-term dangerous effect on our skin and/or our health.

Cosmetics actually still come with lead in them.

What makes that worse is that lead is not shown as an ingredient. As a matter of fact, most cosmetic makers actually hide the ingredients of their products from consumers because they don't want to expose the truth of what's in these high profit items.

The FDA, the governmental approval agency for cosmetics as well as for food and drugs, is nothing if not consistent. The FDA has no problem approving heavy metals and other chemicals in cosmetics that have shown to be carcinogens (that is, cancer-linked). The list of approved items is shocking:

- Parabens
- Triclosan
- Ethoxylates
- Diethanolamine
- Phthalates

These and other dangers come in name-brand products. I'm not talking about only the cheap stuff here.

Your Skin

Your skin is the largest organ in your body. You know that your skin has thousands and thousands of pores. These are small holes, where molecules can go in as well as come out. Your skin is an absorbing organ. Chemicals are not always bad, but all chemicals in all cosmetics, run the risk of entering your system.

Your skin is worth a little extra effort. When you choose cosmetics be sure to read the ingredients. Do your homework and learn what is considered healthy and what is considered dangerous. In general, you should buy cosmetics that are as simple and natural as possible. You don't really need extra junk to be beautiful. As a matter of fact, apple cider vinegar and coconut oil are both wonderful for your skin and hair when you learn how to use them properly.

In a dramatic show of the dangers, the FDA in 2010 tested 22 popular red lipsticks that were currently sold on the market. *Every single one of those 22 lipsticks contained lead.* Lead is a neurotoxin. Lead is a dangerous neurotoxin. I feel the need to repeat the findings: all 22 lipsticks, tested by the FDA, contained lead.

The FDA did nothing except to say that they are not charged with regulating lead in cosmetics. They made it clear that they only regulate the colors, not the toxins that are added to the products. A lot of help they are.

These lipsticks were name brands, well-known brands, some of which I will now name: *Cover Girl, Revlon,* and *L'Oreal.* In their defense, the way the lead gets into these products was explained by the Personal Care Products Council – a pro cosmetic group with financial ties to the industry – who said:

> *Because lead is found naturally in air, water, and soil, it may also be found at extremely low levels as a trace contaminant in the raw ingredients used in formulating cosmetics, just as it is in many thousands of other products.*

Really?

That's not what the *Campaign for Safe Cosmetics*'s spokesperson, Stacy Malkan fully believed. She said this:

> *The lead found in Cover Girl Incredifull Lipcolor Maximum Red was 34 times higher than the lead found in the lowest scoring lipstick, Avon's Ultra Color Rich Cherry Jubilee. Clearly, the manufacturers are capable of doing better.*

Florida's Department of Health stated this in a report on lead poisoning: "There is *no* safe level of lead in blood." I tend to agree.

I want to repeat that your skin absorbs. But not only that, some studies suggest that the average female inadvertently consumes about 4 pounds of lipstick over the course of her life. Four pounds! This is done through eating, sipping tea, licking of the lips, kissing, and so on. Naturally, when you wear lipstick, some does get into the mouth.

Shampoo Isn't Any Exception

In an article named, *The Shocking Truth About Shampoo: Why I Haven't Shampooed in Seven Years*[86], Lea Harris discusses that when she had a baby, she began to worry about her newborn and started looking into the baby lotions and shampoos to see what they contained:

> *"I never did buy that bottle of Johnson's & Johnson's. Especially after finding out the "tear-free" versions contain formaldehyde which prevents tears by numbing the eyes – not because it was gentle and chemical-free!*
>
> *"It was then I discovered the world of natural alternatives to shampoo, cosmetics, personal care items...and everything else. And I ditched my Suave shampoo for good."*

The Biggest Problem is Sodium Lauryl Sulfate (SLS)

Almost every shampoo that you can buy today contains SLS. SLS, or sodium lauryl sulfate, is made from sulfuric acid, sodium salt, and monododecyl ester. At best, SLS is a skin irritant. But it goes further than that. SLS enters into your heart, brain, and other organs through your skin and scalp where it accumulates and causes long-term damaging effects.

Note: SLS enables our shampoo to lather easily. We all like easy lather don't we? But is it worth it?

Just as so many of today's products do, SLS also causes hormone imbalance. SLS is one of the many products that we are exposed to daily that increases our estrogen levels. While this is horrible for women who already get way too much estrogen from the environment and from the food that we eat such as soy products, it is even more dangerous in boys and men.

Yes, I told you that apple cider vinegar is often overrated. It's not overrated when it comes to hair however and neither is organic virgin coconut oil. Those two products can be extremely nice for your hair. People often combine apple cider vinegar and baking soda to produce clean and shiny hair with just the right amount of softness. Although at first the oil in your scalp may wash out too much because of the effectiveness of the apple cider vinegar and baking soda, your scalp quickly adjusts so give it some time.

Other natural shampoos are available, and you can even make your own. Lye soap wasn't just for Granny up in the Tennessee hills! Homemade lye soap is making a comeback in urban homes as more and more moms and wives are learning about the dangers of almost every shampoo (*and soap*) on the market. Every few months, I make a container full of soap bars for my family. Although it saves money over purchasing soap, I don't do it to save money. I do it to save our health.

What to Do about Cosmetics?

Unfortunately, this problem of cosmetic danger is so widespread it's difficult to pay regular price for any product that may be harmful to us. We must continue to do our homework, and we should do business only with those companies that voluntarily label all of the ingredients in their cosmetics. Vote with our dollars and by telling the beauticians at the cosmetic counters that you will only buy products that are fully labeled.

We have to read websites that promote healthy products and explain why they are healthy and what they use to achieve that. Obviously, some "healthy" cosmetics are going to be less effective and not look as good as others. And the difference almost always is going to be price.

But what is the price of health?

20

A WARNING ABOUT PESTICIDES

If you have read anything else by me, especially similar things on our toxic food supply and the way organizations process and handle our food, you won't be surprised that I have very few good things to say about pesticides.

Having said that, it might surprise you though to find that I am not 100% against pesticides!

If a bug infestation occurs, I see little reason not to get some help getting rid of those bugs. The problem is not a spray-when-needed situation. The problem is that we are growing foods such as genetically modified organism-based foods that are designed with pesticides inside of them to kill bugs from seed to final form of food. While this certainly means that crops can get to the market faster and that we possibly can have more of them, we are eating chemically laced food and by the very definition of pesticide, this chemical is a poison that permeates our bodies from virtually everything that we eat.

According to Sally Fallon, in her milestone book called *Nourishing Traditions*, the average plant crop receives 10 applications of toxic pesticides. This is not just on the crops that are out in the field growing, but from start, original seeds are sprayed with pesticides, and more pesticides are applied throughout the life of the product, including once it is picked and in the storage bins ready to ship to market.

> **Note:** Keep in mind that if you're careful to get organic produce that has no pesticides, but failed to eat healthy meats such as grass-fed beef and free-range chickens, you will still get the pesticides because most meats sold today comes from animals that eat pesticide-laced grains from cradle to grave.

Some Highly Worrisome Products, Including Coffee and Tea

As I mentioned in the 10-Hour Coffee Diet section, coffee and tea are some of the most pesticide-laced products on the planet. I have been careful throughout this book to strongly suggest you begin moving to organic products, but at the same time I've tried to make it clear our budgets and busy lifestyles must always come into play too. Some of us cannot afford to buy 100% organic and some of us don't always have the time to seek out the best foods and drinks to buy.

Still, please make yourself a promise that for the 10-Hour Coffee Diet's coffee, or tea if you go that route, *please* do your best to get an organic version. The coffee is so important in that diet plan, and it's used so much, that the quantity demands that you seek organic. I gave you a few links to good-tasting, organic coffee in those earlier chapters.

Fruits and vegetables are sold in the grocery stores as either "conventional" or "organic." Although having the label organic doesn't always mean as healthy as it probably should be, conventional products are far more likely to be sprayed with pesticides and herbicides as well as the genetically modified.

Some fruits and vegetables are more dangerous from the pesticide used than others. For example, according to a 1993 Environmental Working Group Study, strawberries are sometimes sprayed with 500 pounds of pesticides on *each* acre they are grown on! Peppers are next in line, especially green and red bell peppers, being high in neurotoxic residues from pesticides.

The following list of foods is so bad you should avoid them at all costs in their conventional form:

- Strawberries
- Green and red bell peppers
- Spinach
- Cherries
- Peaches
- Mexican cantaloupe
- Celery
- Apples
- Apricots
- Green beans
- Chilean grapes
- Cucumbers[87]

If the fruit or vegetable is grown in countries other than the USA or the UK, you can be sure that even fewer regulations were in place before the food was grown and shipped. For example, bananas are often treated with benomyl, which is linked to birth defects and chlorpyrifos, which is a neurotoxin.

Grains fall right behind fruits and vegetables. Although I would love to see you reduce the number of grains that you and your family eat, you've got to admit that rice and oatmeal are often tasty in moderation. Sadly, among grains, rice and oats were found to be the most contaminated.

What Can You Do to Reduce Pesticides in Your Food?

Outside of purchasing only organic food you can reduce the effects of pesticides on any conventional produce you get. Wash all of your produce properly to remove pesticides.

One of the preferred ways to do this is to use *Dr. Bonner's Sal Suds* (the best choice), or hydrogen peroxide, or just a teaspoon of plain 5% Clorox bleach mixed in a gallon of water. (Yes, the small residual of Clorox isn't as bad as the pesticides. Plus it virtually all rinses off the outer surface of the skin.) Soak your vegetables and fruit for 10 minutes in the solution and rinse them well under pure water.

By following this simple procedure and being consistent with it, you will reduce virtually all pesticide residues from your produce by almost 100%.

Pregnant Mom's Should Be Doubly Aware

If you are a pregnant mom, or the mother of an infant, keep in mind that toxins such as pesticides will be present in your breast milk if you eat foods that contain those poisons. You, more than anyone else, should be eating organic produce throughout your pregnancy and as long as you breast-feed.

The Pesticide & Parkinson's Disease Link

Researchers have found that people who used the popular types of pesticides known as paraquat and rotenone are two and a half times as likely to develop Parkinson's disease.

Yahoo News reported this:

> *Rotenone directly inhibits the function of the mitochondria, the structure responsible for making energy in the cell ... Paraquat increases production of certain oxygen derivatives that may harm cellular structures. People who used these pesticides or others with a similar mechanism of action were more likely to develop Parkinson's disease.*[88]

The big problem with pesticides, herbicides, and fungicides, is that they are neurotoxins and disrupt our neurological systems, including our brains. While it is true that we eat cheaper food because of these neurotoxins, we pay a bigger price with our health.

As I've said earlier, we cannot escape all of this. Sometimes admit it: it's great to just go down to the corner hamburger shop and order a big burger, fries and a shake. Almost certainly, those things are loaded with pesticides, GMOs, high fructose corn syrup, and more chemicals than actual food. But they do taste good, and they make a nice reward once in a while.

The problem is not that we sometimes eat this kind of food and the problem is not that we sometimes buy non-organic produce. The problem is that we, as consumers worldwide, almost always buy the conventional foods that are unhealthy for us, and that are loaded with pesticides, herbicides, and fungicides. Diseases such as Parkinson's disease, and other neurological related diseases, as well as obesity, diabetes, and so many other health issues appear to be directly related to a tainted food supply.

We must begin to watch what we eat, not so much for the calories, but for the source of the food. We must eat more real food. Real food grown by local farmers and our communities is harder to find, but in the long run you may realize these are actually cheaper products! If you find a good source of grass fed beef, where the farmer or rancher did not use grains loaded with pesticides from cradle to grave, you and your family could buy half or a whole cow one or two times and save enough money over the grocery store's price of meat to buy a deep freezer to store your healthy meat in!

Bioaccumulation is the Real Problem

What about the long-term problems with pesticides, herbicides, and fungicides? The problem is not just from a single item that's been sprayed. Dr. Mercola clarifies what's really happening to us:

> *The real problem is something called bioaccumulation.*
>
> *Bioaccumulation means that once these toxins are dumped onto plants and soil, they are very hard to get rid of. Each year tons and tons of these poisons are sprayed on farms, which then run off through the soil into streams and rivers, and eventually these poisons end up in lakes or underground aquifers.*
>
> *These aquifers and lakes feed our water supplies, and some drain into other rivers that reach our oceans.*
>
> *The damage from this continual and massive toxic runoff is very hard to undo. This genie is particularly hard to put back into the proverbial bottle.*[89]

Bioaccumulation Gets Worse!

If that all wasn't bad enough, listen to what Dr. Mercola says happens inside *us:*

> *These man-made neurotoxic chemicals also bio-accumulate in the human body, as they resist breaking down in water and also accumulate and store in fat, where they can remain for long periods of time.*

> *In short, this means your body has a very hard time getting rid of them once they enter it. The link to Parkinson's disease is no doubt caused by a bioaccumulation in brain cells, specifically in the neurons charged with producing dopamine.*
>
> *This is why you don't get Parkinson's disease from eating one piece of pesticide-laden fruit. And why it is so difficult to link this and other degenerative neurological diseases to a single source or cause. It takes years of exposure to reach the disease state, although exposure to massive amounts of these chemicals will produce something called rapid onset Parkinson's, which is another powerful clue to the true nature of these neurotoxins.*
>
> *You see, once enough of these toxic chemicals get into a cell, they disrupt its function. Rotenone inhibits mitochondrial function, while Paraquat increases production of oxygen derivatives.*
>
> *In other words, once enough of these chemicals get into your blood stream, they deposit in the fat inside your brain and begin causing brain damage.*

Omega 3 Can Help

Omega 3 healthy fats found in supplements, such as the Twinlab liquid cod liver oil I talked about earlier in the book, help to protect us at our cellular levels from damage associated with environmental toxins.

About the only kind of fish that we know for sure that has a high amount of Omega 3's and is low or has no Mercury is wild Alaskan salmon. If however you don't eat a lot of wild Alaskan salmon you must supplement with a good Omega 3 fish or cod liver oil. Doing so will help ward off and even reverse some negative health effects that we get in our food supply as a result of pesticides, herbicides, and fungicides that are so common today.

CONCLUSION

Now that you are finished reading the 10-Hour Coffee Diet, the time to start is immediately. As you'll soon see and experience, it's not hard or time-consuming. You'll quickly realize it is a very simple, breakthrough, diet strategy that will revolutionize how people improve their health, increase their energy levels, and lose weight... not only immediately, but over the long term as well.

We gave you a lot to think about. We built in a flexibility to allow you to fit the diet to your personal needs and schedule. This is *not* a "one-size-fits-all" diet that is restrictive and mentally and emotionally draining to do. You are free to go on and off the diet at your convenience for the rest of your life. It's not something you have to do daily, if you don't want to. You might not believe it now, but you also won't feel starved, either.

We showed you that you actually save money while doing the diet... while adding in organic foods. Who doesn't like saving money? Who doesn't like saving time, too! It takes no more than 5 minutes to make a 10-Hour Coffee Diet coffee.

Most people will experience noticeable weight loss, energy improvement, and possible cues that their health's improving within 1 week of doing the 10-Hour Coffee Diet each day. If you are not one of them, please don't lose confidence in the plan. Stick with the plan. This is a flexible, long term, plan. Our goal isn't for you to lose 5 to 10 pounds in the first week (a lot of you will). We all like quick results, but we believe success for you is a long term health and body transformation that takes place over a period of a few months... and then you being able to easily maintain the improved you for the rest of your life while using the 10-Hour Coffee Diet as you see fit.

Good luck and we hope to hear about your weight loss and health transformation!

Sincerely,
Jennifer Jolan and Rich Bryda

REFERENCES

[1] "*Coffee Drinking Statistics*" from The Statistic Brain, http://www.statisticbrain.com/coffee-drinking-statistics/

[2] "*Coffee Taster's Flavor Wheel*," Specialty Coffee Association, http://www.scaa.org/?page=resources&d=scaa-flavor-wheel

[3] Studeville, George. "*Caffeine Addiction Is a Mental Disorder, Doctors Say*." National Geographic. Jan. 15, 2010. http://news.nationalgeographic.com/news/2005/01/0119_050119_ngm_caffeine.html

[4] "*Coffee is the Number One Source of Antioxidants*," http://www.eurekalert.org/pub_releases/2005-08/acs-cin081905.php

[5] "*A Whiff of Coffee Can Wake You Up*," http://www.livescience.com/2614-whiff-coffee-wake.html

[6] "*Coffee drinking associated with lower risk for alcohol-related liver disease*," http://www.eurekalert.org/pub_releases/2006-06/jaaj-cda060806.php

[7] "*Coffee and Tea May Contribute to a Healthy Liver*," Science Daily, http://www.sciencedaily.com/releases/2013/08/130816153019.htm

[8] "*Hold the Diet Soda? Sweetened Drinks Linked to Depression, Coffee May Lower Risk*," http://www.aan.com/PressRoom/home/GetDigitalAsset/10430

[9] "*Coffee drinking tied to lower risk of suicide*," http://news.harvard.edu/gazette/story/2013/07/drinking-coffee-may-reduce-risk-of-suicide-by-50/

[10] *"A Cup of Joe May Help Some Parkinson's Disease Symptoms,"* http://www.aan.com/pressroom/home/pressrelease/1096

[11] "*Why coffee drinking reduces the risk of Type 2 diabetes*," http://www.acs.org/content/acs/en/pressroom/presspacs/2012/acs-presspac-march-14-2012/why-coffee-drinking-reduces-the-risk-of-type-2-diabetes.html

[12] "*Increased Caffeine Intake Is Associated with Reduced Risk of Basal Cell Carcinoma of the Skin*," http://cancerres.aacrjournals.org/content/72/13/3282

[13] "*High Blood Caffeine Levels in Older Adults Linked to Avoidance of Alzheimer's Disease*," http://www.sciencedaily.com/releases/2012/06/120604142615.htm

[14] "*A smart way to start the day*," http://www.cnn.com/2006/HEALTH/01/11/caffeine.smarter/

[15] "*How Coffee Can Galvanize Your Workout*," http://well.blogs.nytimes.com/2011/12/14/how-coffee-can-galvanize-your-workout/?_r=0

[16] Adapted from *Journal of Food Science*, 2010; Pediatrics, 2011; *USDA National Nutrient Database for Standard Reference*, Release 23, 2010; Journal of Analytical Toxicology, 2006; Starbucks, 2011; McDonald's, 2011, Sizes are listed in fluid ounces (oz.) and milliliters (mL), Caffeine is listed in milligrams (mg).

---

[17] *"Intermittent fasting and high intensity fitness boost HGH,"* http://www.naturalnews.com/034704_intermittent_fasting_fitness_HGH.html

[18] *"Study finds routine periodic fasting is good for your health, and your heart,"* http://www.eurekalert.org/pub_releases/2011-04/imc-sfr033111.php

[19] *"Forthcoming study explores use of intermittent fasting in diabetes as cardiovascular disease,"* http://www.eurekalert.org/pub_releases/2013-04/sp-fse042613.php

[20] http://drjoelrobbins.com/

[21] *"Influence of the feeding frequency on nutrient utilization in man: consequences for energy metabolism,"* http://www.ncbi.nlm.nih.gov/pubmed/1905998

[22] *"Compared with nibbling, neither gorging nor a morning fast affect short-term energy balance in obese patients in a chamber calorimeter,"* http://www.ncbi.nlm.nih.gov/pubmed/11319656

[23] *"Burn Away Fat Cells With This Simple Eating Trick,"* http://fitness.mercola.com/sites/fitness/archive/2012/05/04/fasting-effects-on-human-growth-hormone.aspx

[24] *Oil Pulling for a Brighter Smile and Better Health,* http://www.coconutresearchcenter.org/article%20oil%20pulling.htm

[25] *Coconut Oil Offers Hope for Alzheimer's, Parkinson's, and ALS,* http://coconutoil.com/coconut-oil-offers-hope-for-alzheimers-parkinsons-and-als/

[26] *"Coconut Oil and Diabetes,"* http://coconutoil.com/diabetes/

[27] *Antimicrobial Property of Lauric Acid Against Propionibacterium Acnes: Its Therapeutic Potential for Inflammatory Acne Vulgaris*, J Invest Dermatol, Apr, 2009, http://www.ncbi.nlm.nih.gov/pubmed/19387482?ordinalpos=3&itool=EntrezSystem2.PEntrez.Pubmed.Pubmed_ResultsPanel.Pubmed_DefaultReportPanel.Pubmed_RVDocSum

[28] *In vitro antimicrobial properties of coconut oil on Candida species in Ibadan, Nigeria, J Med Food,* Jun, 2007, http://www.ncbi.nlm.nih.gov/sites/entrez?Db=pubmed&Cmd=ShowDetailView&TermToSearch=17651080&ordinalpos=1&itool=EntrezSystem2.PEntrez.Pubmed.Pubmed_ResultsPanel.Pubmed_RVDocSum

[29] *Gluten-free Ketogenic Diet with MCTs Reverses Autism and Eliminates Seizures, Journal of Child Neurology,* http://jcn.sagepub.com/content/early/2013/05/09/0883073813488668.abstract

[30] *"Remove Stubborn Stickers and Glue with Coconut Oil and Baking Soda,"* Lifehacker.com, http://lifehacker.com/remove-stubborn-stickers-and-glue-with-coconut-oil-and-511144764

[31] Robert Lustig, http://profiles.ucsf.edu/robert.lustig

[32] *"MCT Oil: Is it the Ultimate Way to Burn Fat?"*, http://www.bodybuilding.com/fun/issa23.htm

[33] *"Coconut Oil Benefits: When Fat Is Good For You,"* http://www.huffingtonpost.com/dr-mercola/coconut-oil-benefits_b_821453.html

[34] *"The Raw Truth About Milk,"* by Dr. William Campbell Douglas, http://www.amazon.com/The-Raw-Truth-About-Milk/dp/9962636736

[35] *"Two 'Forbidden Foods' That Can Give You Instant Energy,"* http://articles.mercola.com/sites/articles/archive/2012/12/31/top-10-healthiest-foods.aspx

[36] "*About Our Ghee*," http://www.ancientorganics.com/about-our-ghee/

[37] "*Drinking Protein Shakes: How They Can Help You Build Muscle*," http://www.fitday.com/fitness-articles/fitness/strength-training/drinking-protein-shakes-how-they-can-help-you-build-muscle.html#b

[38] "*Research shows superiority of whey protein*," from News Medical, http://www.news-medical.net/news/20131116/Research-shows-superiority-of-whey-protein.aspx?utm_source=rss&utm_medium=rss&utm_campaign=research-shows-superiority-of-whey-protein

[39] "*Medical Ozone and Cancer*," http://oxygenmedicine.com/cancerandozone.html

[40] "*Parabens... the mock estrogen! Why to avoid them at all costs!*," Healthy You, Healthy Family, http://healthyyouhealthyfamily.wordpress.com/2012/08/15/parabens-the-mock-estrogen-why-to-avoid-them-at-all-costs/

[41] "*Is This the Most Dangerous Food for Men?*", http://www.menshealth.com/nutrition/soys-negative-effects

[42] "*5 Reasons High Fructose Corn Syrup Will Kill You*," by Mark Hyman, M.D., http://drhyman.com/blog/2011/05/13/5-reasons-high-fructose-corn-syrup-will-kill-you/

[43] "*Sleep: The Unsung Hero Of Fat Loss*," http://www.bodybuilding.com/fun/sleep-unsung-hero-fat-loss.htm

[44] "*Is It healthy to Skip Breakfast?*", Dr. Joseph Mercola, M.D., http://fitness.mercola.com/sites/fitness/archive/2012/05/04/fasting-effects-on-human-growth-hormone.aspx

[45] "Death by Medicine: Hospital Death Toll Alarming," http://www.laleva.org/eng/2004/05/death_by_medicine_hospital_death_toll_alarming.html

[46] "*Benefit of drinking green tea: The proof is in -- drinking tea is healthy, says Harvard Women's Health Watch*," http://www.health.harvard.edu/press_releases/benefit_of_drinking_green_tea

[47] "What is Leptin?", http://www.news-medical.net/health/What-is-Leptin.aspx

[48] Lindlahr, 1914: USDA 1963 and 1997

[49] "*Vegetables without Vitamins*," *Life Extension Magazine,* March 2001

[50] http://www.aglabs.com/

[51] "*What 'Brain Food' Actually Does for Your Brain*," http://lifehacker.com/5899379/what-brain-food-actually-does-for-your-brain

[52] "*Integrative Psychiatry Inc: Alternative Mental Health Treatment*," http://www.integrativepsychiatry.net/

[53] "*Myelin*," http://www.nationalmssociety.org/about-multiple-sclerosis/what-we-know-about-ms/what-is-ms/myelin/index.aspx

[54] "*The Weston Price Organization,*" http://www.westonaprice.org/

[55] *To Your Good Health, Dr. Al Sears, MD*

[56] *Oil Pulling for a Brighter Smile and Better Health,* http://www.coconutresearchcenter.org/article%20oil%20pulling.htm

[57] *Coconut Oil Offers Hope for Alzheimer's, Parkinson's, and ALS*, http://coconutoil.com/coconut-oil-offers-hope-for-alzheimers-parkinsons-and-als/

[58] Coconut Oil and Diabetes, http://coconutoil.com/diabetes/

[59] *Antimicrobial Property of Lauric Acid Against Propionibacterium Acnes: Its Therapeutic Potential for Inflammatory Acne Vulgaris*, J Invest Dermatol, Apr, 2009, http://www.ncbi.nlm.nih.gov/pubmed/19387482?ordinalpos=3&itool=EntrezSystem2.PEntrez.Pubmed.Pubmed_ResultsPanel.Pubmed_DefaultReportPanel.Pubmed_RVDocSum

[60] *In vitro antimicrobial properties of coconut oil on Candida species in Ibadan, Nigeria*, *J Med Food*, Jun, 2007, http://www.ncbi.nlm.nih.gov/sites/entrez?Db=pubmed&Cmd=ShowDetailView&TermToSearch=17651080&ordinalpos=1&itool=EntrezSystem2.PEntrez.Pubmed.Pubmed_ResultsPanel.Pubmed_RVDocSum

[61] *Gluten-free Ketogenic Diet with MCTs Reverses Autism and Eliminates Seizures*, *Journal of Child Neurology*, http://jcn.sagepub.com/content/early/2013/05/09/0883073813488668.abstract

[62] http://www.consumerfreedom.com/2011/03/4397-pulling-the-curtains-on-another-cspi-scare-campaign/

[63] *Coconut Oil and Alzheimer's: Is the Low-Fat Diet and Cholesterol-Lowering Drugs Part of the Problem?*, http://coconutoil.com/coconut-oil-alzheimers/

[64] *What is Extra-Virgin Olive Oil?,* http://www.oliveoiltimes.com/extra-virgin-olive-oil

[65] *Virgin Coconut Oil,* http://www.tropicaltraditions.com/what_is_virgin_coconut_oil.htm

[66] www.TropicalTraditions.com

[67] *The Truth about Coconut Water*, http://www.webmd.com/food-recipes/features/truth-about-coconut-water?page=2

[68] *Coconut Oil Can Promote Wait Loss by Increasing Metabolism Naturally, August, 2009, NaturalNews,* http://www.naturalnews.com/026808_oil_coconut.html

[69] *Journal of Agricultural and Food Chemistry*, August, 2012, http://www.ncbi.nlm.nih.gov/pubmed/22866697

[70] *Enhancement of muscle mitochondrial oxidative capacity and alterations in insulin action are lipid species dependent: potent tissue-specific effects of medium-chain fatty acids*, *Diabetes*, 2010, May - http://www.ncbi.nlm.nih.gov/pubmed/19720794?dopt=Abstract

[71] *Medium-chain Triglyceride Ketogenic Diet, An Effective Treatment for Drug-resistant Epilepsy and A Comparison with Other Ketogenic Diets*, *Biomed*, Jan, 2013. http://www.ncbi.nlm.nih.gov/pubmed/23515148

[72] *Effects of Dietary Coconut Oil on the Biochemical and Anthropometric Profiles of Women Presenting Abdominal Obesity*, July, 2009, http://www.ncbi.nlm.nih.gov/pubmed/19437058

[73] De Lourdes et al. (2007). *Effects of coconut oil on testosterone-induced prostatic hyperplasia in Sprague-Dawley rats, The Journal of Pharmacy & Pharmacology*, 59(7), 995-999.

[74] *The Surprising Health Benefits of Coconut Oil,* http://www.doctoroz.com/videos/surprising-health-benefits-coconut-oil

[75] Kaunitz, H. 1986. Medium chain triglycerides (MCT) in aging and arteriosclerosis. *J Environ Pathol Toxicol Oncol* 6(3-4):115.

[76] *Coconut Oil and Heart Disease*, http://www.coconutresearchcenter.org/article10132.htm

[77] Li Q, Estes JD, Schlievert PM, Duan L, Brosnahan AJ, Southern PJ, Reilly CS, Peterson ML, Schultz-Darken N, Brunner KG, Nephew KR, Pambuccian S, Lifson JD, Carlis JV, Haase AT. *"Glycerol monolaurate prevents mucosal SIV transmission."* Nature. 2009 Apr 23;458(7241):1034-8

[78] *Coconut Oil Could Combat Tooth Decay,* September, 2012, http://www.bbc.co.uk/news/health-19435442

[79] http://www.naturalnews.com/cancer.html

[80] "*The Weston Price Organization,*" http://www.westonaprice.org/

[81] http://www.livestrong.com/article/457165-normal-daily-sugar-consumption/

[82] http://www.EarthClinic.com

[83] "*Choosing the Right Cinnamon,*" http://www.drfuhrman.com/library/choosing_the_right_cinnamon.aspx

[84] "*Cinnamon Improves Glucose and Lipids of People With Type 2 Diabetes,*" http://care.diabetesjournals.org/content/26/12/3215.long

[85] "*The Benefits of BCAAs,*" http://www.poliquingroup.com/ArticlesMultimedia/Articles/Article/791/The_Benefits_of_BCAAs.aspx

[86] http://www.nourishingtreasures.com/index.php/2012/01/16/the-shocking-truth-about-shampoo-why-i-havent-shampooed-in-seven-years/

[87] Sally Fallon, *Nourishing Traditions*

[88] *Yahoo News, February, 2011,* http://news.yahoo.com/s/afp/20110211/ts_alt_afp/healthusdisease%3B_ylt%3DAts4DL42QJIg0ue7chmTBqis0NUE%3B_ylu%3DX3oDMTFpdmNuNWtoBHBvcwMzOQRzZWMDYWNjb3JkaW9uX21vc3RfcG9wdWxhcgRzbGsDdXNzdHVkeWxpbmtz

[89] http://articles.mercola.com/sites/articles/archive/2011/03/01/us-study-links-pesticides-to-parkinsons-disease.aspx

Made in the USA
San Bernardino, CA
21 September 2017